FOURTH EDITION

Everygirl

Derek Llewellyn-Jones
Suzanne Abraham

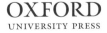

OXFORD
UNIVERSITY PRESS

OXFORD
UNIVERSITY PRESS

253 Normanby Road, South Melbourne, Victoria 3205, Australia

Oxford University Press is a department of the University of Oxford.
It furthers the University's objective of excellence in research, scholarship,
and education by publishing worldwide in

Oxford New York

Auckland Bangkok Buenos Aires Cape Town Chennai
Dar es Salaam Delhi Hong Kong Istanbul Karachi Kolkata
Kuala Lumpur Madrid Melbourne Mexico City Mumbai Nairobi
São Paulo Shanghai Taipei Tokyo Toronto

OXFORD is a trade mark of Oxford University Press
in the UK and in certain other countries

Copyright © 1986, 1992, 1998, 2003 Derek Llewellyn-Jones and Suzanne Abraham
First published 1986
Second edition 1992
Third edition 1998
Fourth edition 2003

National Library of Australia
Cataloguing-in-publication data:

Llewellyn-Jones, Derek, 1923–97.
    Everygirl.

    4th ed.
    Includes index.
    ISBN 0 19 551666 4.

    1. Sex instruction for girls. 2. Teenage girls—Health and hygiene.
    3. Teenage girls—Growth. I. Suzanne Abraham. II. Title.

612.661

Typeset by OUPANZS
Printed in Malaysia through The Bookmaker Pty Ltd

Contents

Acknowledgments

The authors and publishers would like to thank the following for granting permission to reproduce copyright material: Anti-Cancer Council of Victoria (p. 217); Austral International Photographic Library (cover and p. 184); Coo-ee Picture Library (pp. 89 and 225); Domestic Violence and Incest Resource Centre (p. 193); Rennie Ellis (p. 103); International Photographic Library (pp. 9, 19, 147, 234, and 246); Photolibrary.com (pp. 29, 73); Victorian Community Council Against Violence (p. 193).

Thanks also to Johnson & Johnson and the Action Centre for Young People for supplying products for photographic purposes (pp. 50 and 167 respectively).

The authors are grateful to the New South Wales Centre for Education and Information on Drugs and Alcohol and the Australian Government Report of the Child and Adolescent Component of the National Survey of Mental Health and Wellbeing 2000 for providing much of the material on which chapter 16 is based. Similar organisations provide information and education on drugs in other Australian states and in the UK. The authors are also grateful for the expert advice of Dr Amanda McBride, Susan Hart, Tess Poland and, Catherine Boyd.

Disclaimer

Introduction

This introduction is for parents as well as for teenage women, so that they can understand our approach to the needs of 'everygirl'. Nearly all of the book is about changes, problems, and events that occur in the teenage years and the experiences of young women as they pass through the years from about 12 to 20.

When we decided to write *Everygirl* we thought that it would help us if we asked teenage women what they wanted to learn. We found that young women asked for information on these main topics:

- the bodily changes that occur during adolescence
- their own body and that of the other sex
- menstruation
- sexual behaviour
- sexually transmitted diseases
- contraception and pregnancy
- nutrition and eating
- anorexia nervosa, bulimia nervosa, and obesity
- drugs
- acne and medical problems that are more common among teenagers than adults.

In response we have written about many, but not all, of the issues that concern teenagers. For example, we have omitted writing about pregnancy because the book *Everywoman* contains this information. We have also written about a few issues that adults have told us their teenage daughters have told them were important.

There are a few matters that perhaps should be mentioned in this introduction, to show the background of the book. These matters—physical changes, independence, and sexuality—are also discussed in greater detail in later chapters. The remaining issues that we have written about are teenage health concerns, both physical and psychological, and drug-taking.

Physical changes

The first matter relates to the bodily changes that occur during the teenage years. Over this period a young woman's body changes from that of a girl to that of a woman. Her breasts grow and become prominent, and her body shape changes from being stick-like to becoming curvaceous, with obvious hips and thighs. These changes result from the release of the female sex hormones, oestrogen and progesterone, from the young woman's ovaries. After menarche her body weight increases and the growth spurt that occurs early in the teenage years slows down. Today, when fashion dictates that women should be slim, many teenage women are concerned that their body shape and weight are not the 'ideal', as decreed by fashion. This can be distressing to young women, and some of them develop an eating disorder.

Independence

Concurrently with her physical development, a teenage woman's opinions and attitudes develop and change as the years pass. She moves from being a girl dependent on her parents for support and nourishment to a relatively or completely independent woman. For some, this transition is easy, but for others, it is a period of apparent conflict, anger, and anxiety as the teenager and her parents find that their relationship is changing. The young woman no longer accepts all of her parents' values and beliefs. She argues. She might be untidy. However, in spite of popular beliefs, most teenage women continue to hold many of their parents' values and want to love their parents and to be loved in return. Differences in values and beliefs between generations have always occurred, but some parents forget how they behaved when they were teenagers. Parents can help to resolve the conflict by explaining to their daughter why they do not want her to behave in a certain way, and seek her cooperation and agreement, rather than simply saying 'Do this, because I tell you to do it'.

Sexuality

During the teenage years, sex becomes an increasingly important topic of conversation between teenagers, and is a source of concern to many parents and teenagers. It is appropriate to write here, as well as later in the book, about sex as it is perceived by teenagers.

When you hear the word sex, what image is conjured up in your mind? Think for a moment. Most people associate the word sex with the image of a couple having sexual intercourse. In other words, they see sex only as a physical activity, an image that is reinforced by many movies and magazine articles. Sex or, more correctly, sexuality is concerned with much more than sexual intercourse, although sexual intercourse is part of sex.

- Sexuality is the sum of a person's knowledge, experiences, attitudes, and behaviour as they relate to being a woman or a man. It includes those ways of behaving towards another person that increase the love between people and make a person feel good. Feelings are more important in sexuality than actions.
- Sexuality involves how you feel towards another person, as much, or more than, how you enjoy making love to another person.
- Sexuality involves sharing experiences with another person.
- Sexuality involves touching and exploring your own and the other person's body to understand the different textures and surfaces, and to share your knowledge.

- Sexuality involves enjoying the sight or the sound or the smell of another person.
- Sexuality involves being concerned about the other person, and learning to respect the other person's beliefs and attitudes to sex.
- Sexuality involves being responsible to the other person and not forcing your beliefs or attitudes on him or her.
- Sexuality involves being able to talk with the other person, to communicate with the other person. Communication involves more than just talking. It involves listening to what the other person has to say. It means trying to understand what the other person is saying. It means responding.

Nowdays parents believe that their sons and daughters, should learn about sex. Although 90 to 95 per cent of parents believe they are the most appropriate source of information, studies from Australia, the UK, and the USA show that one in six teenagers have not received any sex education from their parents. Parents are sometimes ill-informed about sexuality, or are too shy to answer the questions that their children and teenagers might ask.

Canadian and American parents believe schools should provide courses in sex education as part of personal development courses. They supported instruction at all ages, particularly at high school, and proposed increasing the time provided to enable a greater variety of topics to be covered. Surveys in Australia confirm these findings, with more than 80 per cent of adults believing that education in human sexuality should be provided in schools.

Any opposition to sexuality education is sincere but misguided, because many of the beliefs of those opposing sex education are wrong. Surveys in Australia show that:

- Nearly every teenager surveyed felt a need for sex education.
- Only three in four teenagers felt they had received adequate sex education.
- More than 40 per cent of teenagers obtain their first information about sex from their friends, about 40 per cent from teachers, 15 per cent from parents, and 5 per cent from others.

- Sex education at school does not encourage teenagers to experiment with sex.

Those surveyed believed that:

- Sex education should teach that a person's behaviour should be related to other aspects of her (or his) life and to her (or his) moral, religious, and ethical feelings.
- Sex education should include relationships, parenthood and values.
- Sex education should point out how sex is distorted and exploited in our society.
- Sex education should be given with tolerance, with understanding, and with the acceptance that different people behave differently sexually.
- Sex education should stress that sexual exploitation is not acceptable, it is an affront to human dignity.
- Sex education should help teenagers to become more understanding and tolerant of other people's behaviour and opinions.

Chapter One

It's a girl!

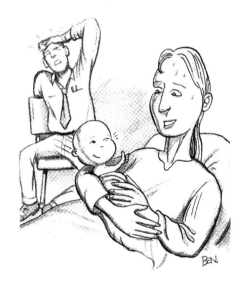

What are little girls made of?
What are little girls made of?
Sugar and spice
And all things nice,
That's what little girls are made of.

Nursery rhyme

When she is young she is called a girl. No one objects to her being called a girl. When she reaches puberty and begins to menstruate can she still be called a girl? Many feminists would say no. To call a teenager a girl is to demean her. She should be called a young woman or just a teenager. Many men call women 'girls', particularly if the man employs the woman in a subordinate job, and this is seen as demeaning. On the other hand, many mature women refer to their friends as girls.

To avoid these problems, in this book we call female children 'girls', and once they have reached puberty we call them 'teenagers' or 'young women'.

How does a person become female?

It is easier to understand the development into a female if the process of conception is described. Conception occurs when a sperm, produced by a man, fertilises an egg (ovum) produced by a woman. The fertilised egg is what develops, ultimately, into a human being.

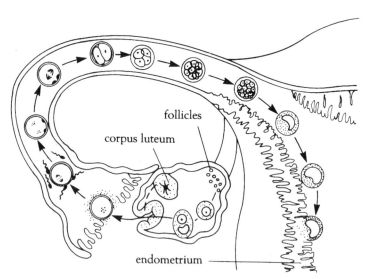

follicles

corpus luteum

endometrium

Figure 1.1 The passage of the ovum from the ovary to fertilisation and implantation.

By the time a girl reaches puberty she has 400,000 eggs in her ovaries. Each egg has a nucleus in its centre, surrounded by tissue. The nucleus carries the genetic information needed to help make a new individual. The egg is surrounded by a soft 'shell', and attached to the outside of the shell is a mantle of cells. Each egg and its mantle of cells in the tissue of the ovaries lies in a tiny 'bag' called a follicle (see figure 1.1).

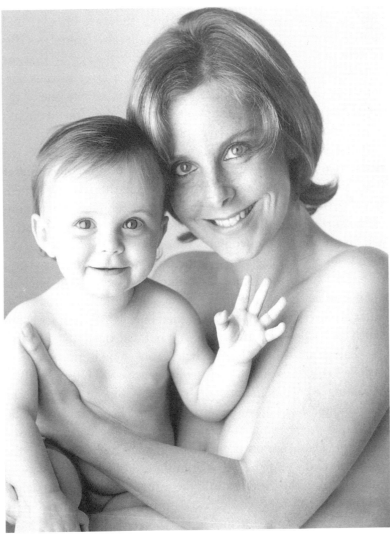

A woman and a woman-to-be.

Each month from puberty at least to the age of 45, between ten and twenty of the 400,000 follicles will grow for about fourteen days and then die. The growth of the selected follicles is due to two hormones secreted by the pituitary gland at the base of the brain. These hormones are called gonadotropic hormones because they stimulate the growth of the gonads (the ovaries and in males the testicles). The first of them is called the follicle-stimulating hormone (FSH) because it acts on the ten to twenty chosen follicles (it is not known how they are chosen) and causes fluid to seep into the follicles. It also stimulates the growth of the mantle of cells that surrounds the egg, so that the follicle becomes bigger. At the same time, a layer of cells surrounding each of the follicles is stimulated to secrete one of the female sex hormones, oestrogen, which enters the woman's blood and acts on many tissues of her body.

For an unknown reason, one (occasionally two) of the stimulated follicles grows more quickly and becomes larger than the others. About halfway between the woman's menstrual periods, this follicle has grown so much that it bulges out of the surface of the ovary. By this time, the amount of oestrogen circulating in the woman's blood has reached a peak. The high level of oestrogen acts on the pituitary gland and causes it to release the second gonadotrophic hormone, called luteinising hormone (LH). This hormone induces the swollen follicle to burst and to release the egg contained in it, which is quickly but gently propelled into the frond-surrounded opening of one of the Fallopian tubes. The follicle from which the egg was expelled collapses and, under the influence of LH, turns yellow, becoming a corpus luteum (or 'yellow' body) and secretes the second female sex hormone, progesterone. Progesterone is vital because it prepares the lining of the uterus to receive a fertilised egg should conception occur. If pregnancy does not occur the corpus luteum and the other stimulated follicles wither away and die. But the next month the process starts again when another ten to twenty follicles start growing. If pregnancy does happen, the corpus luteum grows bigger and secretes more progesterone.

Conception and fertilisation

Conception will occur only if a sperm manages to penetrate the soft 'shell' of the egg (ovum) within forty-eight hours of its expulsion from its follicle.

When a man has sexual intercourse with a woman and ejaculates (comes) in her vagina, about 300 million sperm spurt out of his penis, equal to about a tablespoonful of fluid. When he withdraws his penis from the woman's vagina, most of the fluid containing the sperm seeps out of her vagina, but some remains.

Each sperm is made up of an oval head, which contains the sperm's nucleus; a tubular body, which is the engine of the sperm; and a long tail (see figure 1.2). After ejaculation, the sperm thrash about in the woman's vagina, by the movement of their tails. They cannot penetrate her uterus because the narrow passage that leads through its neck (or cervix) is blocked by a matted network of strands of mucus. Only at the time of ovulation does the mesh of mucus disappear, when it is replaced by spiral channels in the mucus, each just wide enough to fit a sperm.

If the couple has intercourse at the time that the woman ovulates, several million of the sperm ejaculated into her vagina are able to swim up through the twisting channels in the mucus to enter the uterus. Driven by their thrashing tails, a few thousand survive to reach the entrance to the Fallopian tubes. Some of the survivors manage to enter the Fallopian tubes and to swim along them (see figure 1.3). If the sperm have entered the Fallopian tube that contains the newly ovulated egg, a few might manage to reach the egg, which is 1000 times larger than

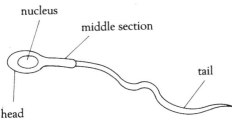

Figure 1.2　A sperm.

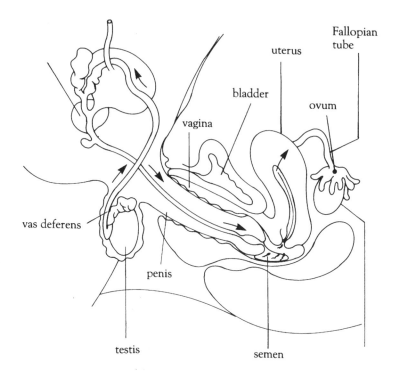

Figure 1.3 The journey of the sperm to fertilise an ovum.

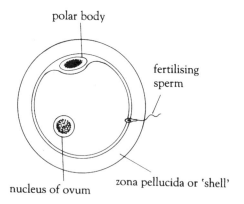

Figure 1.4 Conception occurs when a sperm penetrates the shell of the ovum and fuses with the core genetic material in the ovum.

the sperm (see figure 1.4). One of these sperm might manage to penetrate the soft shell surrounding the egg. If this happens, a change occurs in the shell that prevents any other sperm from penetrating the shell.

The head of the sperm that has managed to enter the substance of the egg then separates from its body and tail, and moves to lie beside the nucleus of the egg. The body and the tail of the sperm dissolve. Inside the egg, the head dissolves, leaving the sperm's nucleus free. At once it fuses with the nucleus of the egg. Conception has occurred.

The fertilised egg develops in the outer part of the Fallopian tube for two or three days, and then it is gently propelled along the tube to reach the cavity of the uterus, where it implants into the lining of the uterus (the endometrium; see figure 1.1).

Not every fertilised egg implants. It is estimated that one in three fails to implant and is discarded by the woman's body.

Pregnancy rates

Pregnancy occurs fairly easily and quickly for 90 per cent of couples who are planning to have a baby. If a couple have regular intercourse at ovulation time, one woman in three will become pregnant in that month. If a couple have sexual intercourse during the time of ovulation each month for a year, nine out of ten couples will achieve their desired pregnancy.

If pregnancy does not occur, the ten to twenty stimulated follicles, including the follicle that has collapsed, die, and the cycle starts again.

Sex determination

The egg and the sperm are called gametes. The nucleus of each contains twenty-three long strands of twisted material called chromosomes. Each chromosome is composed of several thousand genes, like beads on a necklace. The genes contain the bits of information needed to make a new individual.

Every cell in a person's body (with the exception of the gametes) contains forty-six chromosomes; this number is characteristic of the human race. Forty-four of the chromosomes transmit bodily characteristics from parent to child, which is why children tend to resemble their parents. However, not all the characteristics are transmitted, and some are hidden, which is why each person is an individual.

The remaining two chromosomes are the sex chromosomes, which determine whether the person will be female or male. There are two kinds of sex chromosomes. One is called X because of its shape. The other is called Y, also because of its shape.

The gametes—the eggs and the sperm—contain only half the number of chromosomes in their nuclei. Each egg contains twenty-two general chromosomes and one X chromosome. The sperm are different. About half carry twenty-two general chromosomes and one X chromosome, and the other half carry twenty-two general chromosomes and one Y chromosome.

Chance determines which sperm will fertilise the egg. If the fertilising sperm carries an X chromosome, the resulting person

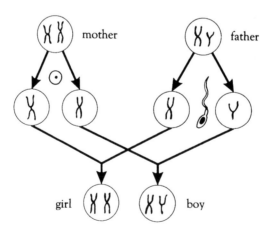

Figure 1.5 Sex determination. An X chromosome from the mother combines with a Y from the father for a boy; an X from the mother combines with an X from the father for a girl.

will be female, because each cell of her body will have twenty-two general chromosomes and one X chromosome from the father and twenty-two general chromosomes and one X chromosome from the mother (see figure 1.5). In this way the number of chromosomes is restored to that found in all humans—forty-six (forty-four general chromosomes and two sex chromosomes).

If the sperm that fertilises the egg carries a Y chromosome, the resulting person will be male, and every cell in his body will contain forty-four general chromosomes and an X and a Y sex chromosome (again giving a total of forty-six).

When the nucleus of the sperm and that of the egg fuse, an exchange of chromosomes occurs. Quite quickly the fused cell divides and then the two new cells divide and the process goes on to form a ball of cells, called a pre-embryo.

Preselecting the sex of the child

Most couples are pleased with the baby whether it is a girl or a boy, but in some cultures it is considered very important for a married couple to have at least one son. A son ensures that the family's name continues. A son gives the father status among his friends. A son gives the family power. This is because, in many societies, men can do many more things than women. Women in such societies are subordinate to men. Women care for children, cook food, fetch water, and garden. Men do exciting things, and they control women. In many societies, when a woman marries she joins her husband's family and is lost to her own family, sometimes never seeing them again. In a few societies, such as the Minangkabau in Sumatra, women are more powerful than men as land is inherited through them.

Because of the common preference to have a son, many couples seek all kinds of supposed methods to achieve a boy child. Sometimes the couple get the son they want, sometimes they do not. None of the methods is uniformly successful.

When it was discovered that the sex of the unborn baby was determined by the father's sperm, some doctors thought they could do better than the magicians and folk medicine experts in helping a couple 'preselect' the sex of their child.

One doctor suggests that as the Y chromosome is smaller than the X chromosome, the sperm carrying a Y chromosome is lighter and more active than the sperm carrying the X chromosome. He believes that the more active sperm travels faster and reaches the egg sooner. He says that if you want a boy you should have intercourse at the time of ovulation, while if you want a girl you should have intercourse two or three days before the time of ovulation and then abstain. He claims success with the method, but no other doctor has been successful with this technique. A more sophisticated method uses the same belief that male-carrying sperm are more active. The scientists argued that if you put a specimen of sperm into a long tube filled with egg white, Y-carrying sperm migrate further and can be collected. The early results of the technique showed that more boys than girls were conceived using the technique, but as more results came in, as many girls as boys were conceived.

All this means that chance, not science, determines the sex of a baby.

Twins

In some women, two follicles grow more rapidly than the other chosen follicles, and two eggs are expelled. If these two eggs are fertilised, the woman will have twins. The twins might both be girls, both boys, or one of each, depending on which kind of sperm has fertilised them. These twins will be 'fraternal' twins, not identical twins. Identical twins occur when a single fertilised egg divides to form two identical eggs, each of which grows into a baby. As both babies have come from the same egg, fertilised by the same sperm, their chromosomes are identical.

Chapter Two

Becoming a girl

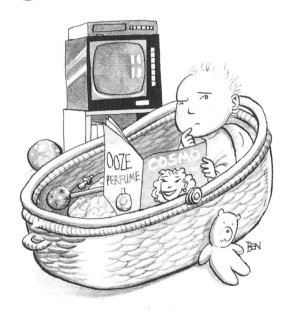

One is not born a woman: one becomes
a woman.

Simone de Beauvoir, The Second Sex

The chromosomal sex of the fetus, described in chapter 1, is only the first, although the most important, stage in the progress of the fetus to become female or male. The sex chromosome status of every body cell, whether XX (female) or XY (male), now influences the second stage of sexual development, the genital sex.

Genital development

This stage starts about six weeks after conception. At this time, when the fetus is only 3 mm long, two ridges of tissue, called gonads, form in the abdomen of the fetus, one on each side of what will become the spinal cord. Almost immediately, millions of cells migrate into the ridges and concurrently two sets of ducts (tubes) form, adjacent to the ridges. If the fetus is chromosomally female, that is, her body cells contain XX sex chromosomes, the cells in the ridges will become egg cells (ova), and will produce the female sex hormone, oestrogen. If the fetus is chromosomally male, that is, his body cells contain XY sex chromosomes, the ridges will turn into testicles, which will secrete the male sex hormone, testosterone, and, after puberty, will produce millions of sperm each day.

Even at this early stage of sexual development, oestrogen and testosterone secreted by the gonads are important because they act on the sets of ducts that were formed. These ducts extend down from the gonads to the genital area of the fetus, which is marked by a tiny knob of tissue. If the fetus is male, the testosterone secreted by its testicles cause one set of the ducts (the female set) to wither away and the male set to grow. These ducts will form the tubes (the vas deferentia) that lead from the testicles through the prostate gland and along the penis. The penis has developed from the tiny knob of tissue.

In the absence of the Y chromosome, the male set of ducts withers away and the female set grows to form the Fallopian tubes, the uterus, and the upper part of the vagina. The lower part of the vagina is formed, later in the pregnancy, by an ingrowth of tissue from the genital area, and the knob of tissue becomes the clitoris.

This process has led to the second stage of sexual development, the genital sex.

Apart from this sexual development, the rest of the fetus develops in the same way, regardless of whether the sex is female or male. This explains why, immediately after a baby has been born, it is impossible to tell whether it is a girl or a boy unless you look at the genitals. If a small penis and a scrotum are visible, the newborn baby is a boy. If a slit is visible, the baby is a girl.

Apart from their genitals, newborn babies look alike at birth and continue looking alike for a few years, but quite quickly their behaviour becomes different.

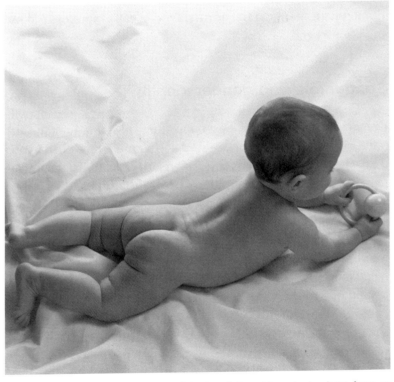

From the back view, it is impossible to distinguish a baby boy from a baby girl.

The seeds for the different behaviour of males and females probably begin before birth. As mentioned above, a male fetus's testicles start secreting small amounts of the male hormone, testosterone, while he is still in his mother's uterus. The testosterone circulates through his body. Some attaches to his brain cells, where the hormone is believed to 'imprint' a pattern of male behaviour, which will show itself after the baby is born. It is not known for certain whether this occurs in humans, but it certainly does in some other mammals. For example, in an experiment, female rhesus monkey fetuses were given injections of testosterone. The behaviour of these female monkeys after birth was indistinguishable from that of male monkeys of a similar age and dissimilar from the behaviour of female monkeys. The injected monkeys were more active, they played rough and tumble games, they chased and threatened other monkeys, all of which the normal female baby monkeys did far less often.

Gender role and gender identity

Even if this male behaviour imprinting exists in humans, its influence is far less important in determining a boy's behaviour than the way in which parents, relatives, and friends treat female and male children, almost from the moment of birth, although the effect of this on the infant's behaviour does not appear for nearly a year.

Child psychologists who study human behaviour have found that human children, from about the age of nine months, begin behaving in specific ways by imitating those around them and responding to the way their parents and relatives want them to behave. Many parents behave differently to their baby from the time of its birth, depending on its sex, but the baby only starts responding differently at about nine months of age. The baby girl learns very quickly that if she behaves in a way in which her parents want her to behave, she will be praised and rewarded. A boy baby learns the same lesson.

The process of learning to behave in the way in which other people expect the infant to behave is called 'role taking', and, in the case of an infant, the parents start forming a 'gender role' for the baby, which the baby rapidly learns to adopt. A gender role is demonstrated by everything a person does or says to indicate to others that she is a girl or he is a boy.

If you observe small babies, you will find that they show no awareness of their gender, at least until they are about nine months old. And, during these months, boy babies and girl babies do not show any differences in their behaviour.

After the age of nine months the baby becomes more mobile, starts exploring, and begins to receive a wider variety of information from its observations. It begins to learn its gender role as more and more bits of information are stored in its brain cells. The baby now begins to look at and assess women and men differently. For example, the baby might observe that its mother is usually the person who looks after its needs, while its father and other males are usually more distant, less nurturant, and perhaps seem physically stronger and more powerful.

By the age of 2, the child has learnt to identify an increasingly large number of objects by observation and by learning. For example, a girl learns that a furry object with a small face and four legs, and which purrs, is called a cat. And if she plays with the cat she learns more—perhaps that it scratches.

Although the 2-year-old girl can identify a cat, she is still learning to distinguish men from women. She learns that women and men wear different clothes, that they have different hairstyles and might or might not have hair on their face, and that they have different smells. The child also learns by watching and listening as males and females discuss each other. The child learns that women and men seem to do different things. She may learn that women are likely to spend more time at home, caring for children, cooking, keeping the house tidy. She learns that men tend to do certain things that require strength or mechanical skills.

In these ways the child learns that women and men do different things, in other words have different 'gender roles'.

But at this stage the girl has not learnt that she is female; in other words, she has not developed a gender identity. A gender identity develops when a person becomes aware that she is female or he is male. This awareness occurs at about the age of 3, and seems to coincide with the child's ability to use language properly. When this occurs the girl can say with conviction: 'I am a girl.' She knows that she is not a boy and has some idea of the ways in which a boy is different. Within the next year, a girl is able to identify other children as girls or boys; and by the age of 5, at the latest, believes that her gender identity is firm and unchangeable. (A very few boys and girls fail to have this fixed gender identity and might later become transsexual.)

Traditional gender roles

The importance of having exclusive gender roles for women and men has diminished in the last fifty years. Insistence on clearly defined gender roles can be disadvantageous to females. In our society the gender roles are still generally those of non-industrial societies (although this is gradually changing). In many such societies there was a clear separation of male and female roles. The men were hunters; the women gave birth to and nurtured their many children, breast-feeding for two years or longer, gathered fruits and grains, and cooked. Although the tribe depended on the women for most of its food, women usually had less power. Women were excluded from decision-making and 'important' events, except for the mysteries of menstruation and childbirth, which were women's secrets.

In pre-industrial societies today, such as those in rural Africa, Asia, and South America, food production and the economic structure are still based on women and men filling different roles. These societies emphasise male aggressiveness and competitiveness and female submission, subordination, and compliance. Such attitudes limit the roles that women and men can play.

Modern gender roles

In Western post-industrial society today, women have more choices. Reliable contraceptive measures have meant that women (and their partners) can choose to have fewer children or to have none at all. The alternatives to the traditional female role (whereby the female stayed at home attending to family and household needs) have meant that more women are able to resume careers after devoting less time to child-rearing or have continued to work in a career (in addition to, or instead of, raising children). There are problems, however, for many women who opt for the less traditional female role.

Even today, many women are disadvantaged in opportunities for jobs. They obtain less interesting jobs, get less pay, achieve lower levels of promotion. This is not due to lack of ability or ambition but to the patriarchal (male-dominated) structure of society. In a male-dominated society, women have to expend more effort, more time, and more skill to achieve a position that a less-qualified man achieves more easily. This biases the competition strongly in favour of a man; it ceases to be true competition. Change is slow.

The lack of success of women in high-status jobs might also be affected by the way in which girls are reared. Females are taught to take orders from authority more easily and comply with them more readily; women are less likely to protest and are slower to become angry, so they are easier to exploit by men and are readier to take less interesting, lower-status jobs. Males are more likely to be verbally and physically aggressive, and they become angry more quickly than females. This might be due to the fact that men produce testosterone, the male sex hormone in the testes: animals that have been castrated when young show much less aggressive behaviour when they become adult than do uncastrated animals. But humans are not animals in this sense, and many psychologists believe that the different ways girls and boys are reared are more influential on the way they behave than are their sex hormones.

As differences in behaviour are reinforced by the different ways the two sexes are reared, it tends to be self-perpetuating. Women brought up to feel inferior might come to believe that they are inferior to men. Even when the work of men and women is of identical quality, women tend to 'put down' that of their own sex and to rate a man's work more highly.

Why women perpetuate their sense of subordination is not an easy question to answer. Anthropologists have found that many repressed minority groups tend to adopt the attitudes of the stronger dominant group towards themselves. Women might do the same by accepting the submissive stereotype and, by this device, are able to escape some of the anxiety that arises if they feel themselves to be oppressed. It is often easier to accept life as it is than to rebel against it.

Some adults fear that any reduction in the differences between the way the sexes look and behave and what they do in sexual encounters, in work, or in play will lead to a destruction of the fabric of society. This is a false fear: equality of opportunity for women in all spheres of activity will not reduce the gender identity of women, but rather will permit women to develop as freer human beings. The reduction in a man's competitiveness and aggression, and the social permission for him to show emotion and affection, will not reduce his male gender identity but will enable him to relate more freely and equally with other human beings, regardless of their sex.

The difference between girls and boys

As mentioned, most scientists now believe that the prenatal influence of the male hormone on the behaviour of a boy child, and its absence in a girl child, is small compared with the socialising influence of parents, relatives, and friends on the growing child. In spite of this knowledge, several myths persist about the behaviour of little girls. The reality of the development and behaviour of little girls is described below.

Most of the differences in the behaviour of little girls and little boys are because they are taught to behave differently.

These lessons are well absorbed by many young women as they approach puberty, by which time they have learnt to be dependent and submissive. They will also have learnt not to be aggressive physically (but that verbal aggression might be permitted).

Little girls: the reality

- Little girls are encouraged to show dependency; this is not permitted to little boys.
- Little girls are not more dependent on those who care for them than are little boys.
- Little girls do not spend longer playing with other children than do little boys.
- Little girls are not more likely to imitate other people than are little boys.
- Little girls are not less able to understand complex ideas than are little boys.
- Little girls are not better at doing repetitive tasks than are little boys.
- Little girls can analyse problems as competently as little boys.
- Little girls are as self-confident as little boys.
- Little girls do not cry more than little boys (at least up to the age of 3, by which time little boys have been taught not to cry).
- Little girls are not more timid or anxious than little boys (at least up to the age of 9, before learned behaviour interferes).
- Little girls are not more helpful to others than are little boys.
- Little girls are encouraged to show emotions; little boys are discouraged from showing emotions.
- Little girls are encouraged to touch and be touched; little boys are discouraged from touching.
- Little girls are discouraged from behaving aggressively, whereas little boys are encouraged to imitate aggressive acts, to indulge in rough and tumble play, and to hit each other.

What causes these differences? One theory is that male children are treated differently from female children, being encouraged to be more aggressive and less compliant. An alternative theory is that there is a 'feminine' gene carried on an X chromosome that causes females to be more compliant, more sensitive, more considerate, and more able to relate to others than males.

Chapter Three

Puberty and adolescence

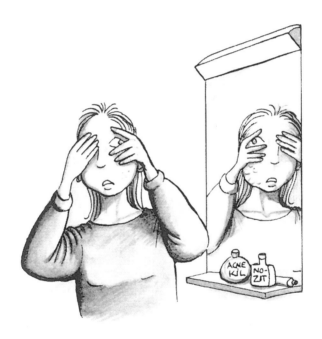

Thank heaven for little girls!
For little girls get bigger every day.
Alan Jay Lerner, 'Thank Heaven for Little Girls'

The word *adolescence* is derived from the Latin word *adolescere*, which means 'to grow up'. *Puberty* comes from the Latin *pubescere*—'to grow hairy'. Today, adolescence is used to describe the period of time from puberty to adulthood, which itself is not readily defined, although most people would define a person as being adult when she or he has reached full physical and emotional development and is able to look after himself or herself efficiently.

Adolescence

The concept of adolescence is fairly recent. Until 150 years ago, most children were assumed to be miniature adults; they developed directly from children to adults, without passing through an intermediate period. At about the age of 12, female children were expected to take part in all the household duties done by women and to learn the skills needed to be a good wife. Male children at about the same age took part in all the work done by the male parent, or were apprenticed to another family to learn a trade.

Only when it was appreciated that a longer period of education produced a more useful person, and when social movements developed to limit the work that teenage children might or might not undertake, did the concept of adolescence become accepted. Allied to this was increasing concern in Western nations about the exploitation to which young people were exposed and their need for adult guidance. Most of these changes applied only to the middle class and to the rich; the poor both in the country and in the towns continued to be exploited.

Today, adolescence is perceived in most countries as an important stage in a person's development. Adolescence can usefully be divided roughly into three stages:
early adolescence (up to about 16 years of age)
mid adolescence (about 15–17)
late adolescence (about 17–19).

> ### Adolescent women
> - Care more for others' feelings and welfare.
> - Are more concerned about gaining social approval and avoiding disapproval.
> - Are more concerned about intimacy.
> - Are more inclined to show shame.
> - Are more concerned about appearance.

Early adolescence

At this stage, the girl is concerned about her rapidly growing body and her appearance. She compares her development with that of other girls of her own age. She becomes concerned about

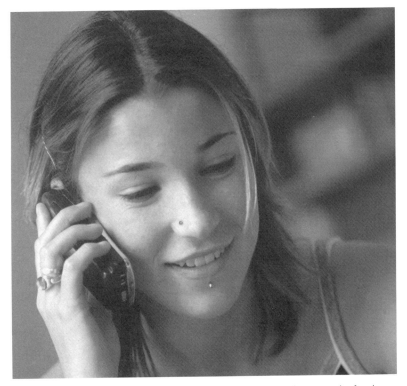

During adolescence, teenagers need to establish their own set of values. Sometimes these are different from their parents' values, but often they are quite similar.

what other people will think of her appearance. If she dislikes her looks she might become moody and anxious. She might sleep poorly. Her sexuality is awakening, and she might have a series of crushes on older people, which for a time are all-absorbing.

Mid adolescence

Sexual attractions to boys become more powerful at this stage, and it becomes as important for a teenager to behave like her peers as for her to accept her parents' values. She resents criticism from adults that she feels is unjustified, and is particularly resentful if her parents appear not to be taking her problems and anxieties seriously. Her fantasy life increases in scope and complexity. Her body image continues to be important. She might experiment with new hairstyles and make-up. She worries about acne.

Late adolescence

The teenager is passing out of the times of confusion. She will generally have achieved an acceptable degree of independence from her parents. She will have made more mature relationships. She will have clearer ideas of what she wants to do in life.

During the three stages of adolescence, a teenage women has several tasks that she needs to deal with in order to become an adult.

First, she has to come to terms with and accept her body and her appearance. Most teenage women are worried about the size and shape of their body or some specific part of their body. Most young women want to achieve the currently fashionable body shape. Of particular importance to many young women is the size of their breasts. Breasts have a potent erotic value, which is emphasised in magazines, films, and TV shows. The fashionable, desired breast size changes over the years, but the breasts themselves continue to be erotically arousing to men, and often to women. Because of the importance of breasts, a number of myths surround them, and some of these myths are listed in the box below.

Myths about breasts

- Women are unconcerned about the size of their breasts.
- Large breasts indicate that the woman is likely to be more interested in sex.
- Women with small breasts are unable to breast-feed successfully.
- Breast-feeding leads to sagging breasts.
- Hair on the area around the nipples indicates that the woman is abnormal.
- All women enjoy having their breasts fondled.
- Women with big breasts are very fertile.

Second, a teenage woman has to come to terms with her sexual feelings, needs, and desires; coming to terms with them is a major task during adolescence.

Third, a teenage woman must achieve independence from her parents, at the same time being able to enjoy their company and to seek help from them when needed. Achieving independence can be traumatic to parents and to the young woman herself. Each side must try to understand the concerns of the other, and each has to accept that much of their behaviour seems irrational to the other. When both sides can listen to (but not necessarily agree with) the other's point of view, the task is made less difficult. When they cannot communicate, problems can occur. Dr Rutter, an English psychiatrist who has made many studies of adolescent behaviour, puts this precisely when he writes:

> But perhaps the most striking characteristic of many families with a disturbed adolescent is their inefficient communication, both in the sense that discussion tends to be associated with fruitless disputes, and in the sense that it often fails to give rise to an agreed solution.

Fourth, a teenage woman has to develop a system of values, ideals, and behaviour that are right for her but do not damage the values and ideals of others to any great extent. A few teenagers show antisocial, destructive behaviour, but most find that their values and ideals are not too far removed from those of their parents.

Finally, a teenage women must learn skills and attitudes that will enable her to become financially independent of her parents.

Puberty

Puberty refers more specifically to the time when the visible signs of sexual maturity start. In females, puberty is marked by the onset of menstruation; in males, puberty is not so exactly defined, but is usually identified by the growth of the boy's penis and testicles.

The physical changes that are the visible signs of puberty are due to hormones produced in the girl's body. The changes begin quietly. The first change occurs when a girl is aged about 8.

A gland, called the adrenal gland, which lies in her body like a cap over the top of the kidneys, begins to secrete increasing amounts of a hormone, adrenal androgen. Scientists have not elucidated what this hormone does to the body in a young girl. This adrenal activation is the first of a series of glandular awakenings that occur over the next four or five years, and are most marked in the two years before menstruation starts, that is, the onset of puberty.

All of these glands are controlled by secretions from a key area in the lower part of the brain called the hypothalamus. The hypothalamus secretes and releases hormones, which travel the short distance between it and the pituitary gland. The hormones are called 'releasing hormones' because they induce specialised cells in the pituitary gland to release hormones that act on other glands of the body. In the years before puberty, the first of the pituitary hormones to be released is the growth hormone. This induces body growth and is responsible for the growth spurt that starts in girls about the age of 10 (and rather later in boys). The age at which the growth spurt starts is quite variable. Some girls grow quickly at the age of 9, in other girls the growth spurt is delayed until the age of 14. This means that girls of the same age can vary considerably in their height.

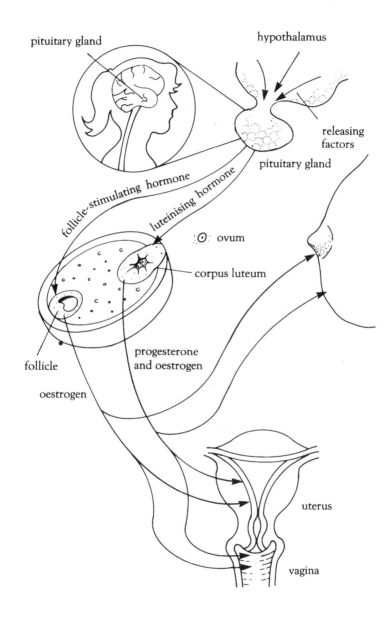

Figure 3.1 The role of hormones during the reproductive years.

A few months after the growth hormone is secreted in increasing quantities, the hypothalamus sends hormonal messages via the gonadotrophic-releasing hormone to the gonadrotrophic cells in the pituitary gland (see figure 3.1). (In reality, the hypothalamus has been sending the hormonal messages for a number of years, but the messages have been of low amplitude.) Now the hormonal pulses are bigger, and they occur more frequently. The effect of these pulses is to induce the pituitary gland to secrete and release follicle-stimulating hormone (FSH) into the blood. As mentioned in chapter 1, the FSH acts on some of the cells of the girl's ovaries to produce the female sex hormone called oestrogen. (In spite of its name, FSH also acts on the cells of a boy's testicles, inducing them to grow and to produce the male sex hormone, testosterone.)

Table 3.1 The physical changes during the teenage years

Age (average)	Body changes
9–10	The bony pelvis begins to grow. Fat begins to be deposited on the hips and thighs so that the body shape begins to change. The nipples begin to bud.
10–11	The breasts begin to bud. A small amount of sparse soft hair grows on the skin around the external genitals (the pubic area).
11–14	The breasts increase in size and become conical. The nipple area becomes obvious and darker. The internal genitals begin to grow larger. The vagina might become moist, and some discharge might appear. The pubic hair becomes thicker and curly.
12–15	The breasts become rounded. The nipple area is raised. The hips become rounder, as fat is deposited. The first menstruation occurs (called menarche). The pubic hair is thick, curly, and coarse.
16–17	Body growth stops—you have reached your adult height. The menstrual periods are regular.

Under the stimulus of FSH, the girl's ovaries secrete increasing amounts of oestrogen into the blood, and, over a few years, this converts her body from that of a child to that of a woman. The changes that occur can be listed, and the average age at which they occur has been determined (see table 3.1). However, it must be stressed that these are *average* ages: different girls whose growth and development is normal will experience these changes at different ages.

As well as the physical changes in the body that can be seen by the girl and by her family and friends, oestrogen and androgen (the latter is produced mainly in her ovaries) act on the tissues of the genital tract. The vagina increases in length and is able to be distended, and its walls become thicker. Small amounts of secretions may be detected by the young woman if she feels inside her vagina. Her uterus grows in size, its muscle becoming thicker and stronger, and its lining (the endometrium) developing. The Fallopian tubes become longer and better prepared to receive an egg and help it on its journey into the uterus.

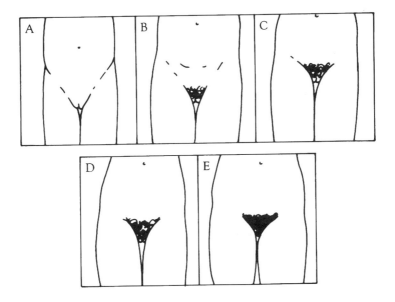

Figure 3.2 The growth pattern of pubic hair. (a) Age 10–11. (b) Age 11–14. (c) Age 12–13. (d) Age 13–15. (e) Adult.

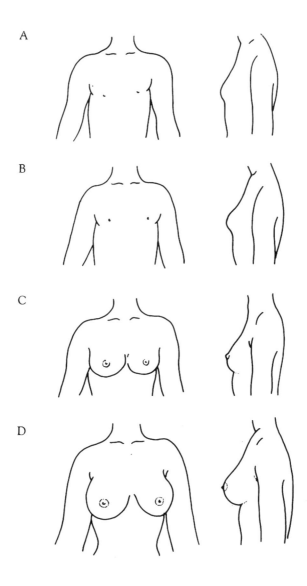

Figure 3.3 Breast development. (a) The beginnings of breast growth. (b) There is more breast tissue. (c) The nipple has a separate outline from the breast. (d) Shape of the adult breast: nipple and breast have the same shape.

Oestrogen also causes the depositing of fat on the young woman's hips (see figure 3.2) as well as the visible growth of the breasts (see figure 3.3). Testosterone is increasingly secreted by the ovaries and is indirectly responsible for the growth of pubic hair (see figure 3.2) and for the increase of muscle mass. The quantity of testosterone secreted in teenage females is much smaller than that secreted by a male's testicles, which is why teenage men have stronger muscles than teenage women. (Testosterone also has the undesired effect of inducing acne, which unfortunately affects more than half of all teenage women. See chapter 14 for more information on acne.)

The hormones secreted by the ovaries prepare the uterus for a possible pregnancy and, once ovulation occurs, a second sex hormone, progesterone, adds to the effect of the uterus (see chapter 1). Once the uterus has responded appropriately to oestrogen, the girl's body has developed sufficiently, and enough fat has been deposited in her tissues, the marker of puberty in girls, the first menstrual period, occurs.

Chapter Four

Menstruation and menstrual problems

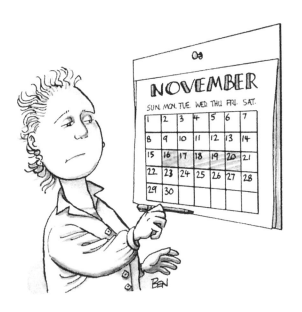

When God was creating women, you'd think He could have shown their fertility a little more conveniently.

Anon.

Menstruation is the periodic red discharge (usually at monthly intervals) from the uterus of a mixture of blood, tissue fluids, and tiny pieces of the lining of the uterus (the endometrium). The amount of blood and tissue fluids in the menstrual discharge varies, but the exact quantities of each cannot be determined by looking at the discharge. Usually a woman menstruates (i.e. has a period) every twenty-six to thirty days, but it is normal for menstruation to occur at intervals from twenty-two to thirty-five days.

Sometimes a woman consults a doctor because she is worried about her periods. The doctor asks questions to try to find out what is worrying her. One of the questions the doctor asks is: 'How often does your period occur?' This might confuse the woman if she wonders whether the question means how many days are there *between* periods, or how many days are there from the beginning of one period to the beginning of the next. In fact, the doctor is asking 'How many days is it from day one of your period to day one of your next period?' so that she or he can calculate the length of the menstrual cycle.

As well as the length of the menstrual cycle, it is usual for a doctor to ask how many days the period lasts and to enquire about the amount of the menstrual discharge. A heavy menstrual discharge, which appears as heavy bleeding, is a common concern in the teenage years. In the first two or three years after periods start, they often occur at longer intervals than later and might occur at irregular intervals. (The reason for this is that the teenage woman is not yet ovulating regularly, and so consequently the hormonal control of the endometrium is not precise.) By the age of 16, most teenagers have regular periods, and they remain regular (unless a pregnancy occurs) until the woman is older than 40 and is approaching the age when women cease to menstruate, in other words, have reached the menopause.

As mentioned above, it is sometimes difficult for a woman to estimate how much blood is lost in the menstrual discharge, as the quantity of blood in the discharge varies, the balance consisting of tissue fluid. In other words, the menstrual discharge might be profuse, but the blood loss is still in the normal range.

Most women lose an average of 30 mL of blood during a period, but it is normal to lose as little as 3 mL or as much as 80 mL. A blood loss of more than 80 mL is excessive and, if the total menstrual discharge is also excessive, might be associated with episodes of 'flooding', when the menstrual discharge seems to pour out of a woman's vagina. If the blood lost in the discharge is considerable and continues for some months, the woman might become anaemic. For this reason, if your periods are very heavy, it would be sensible to visit a doctor.

To try to find out how much blood you are losing, the doctor might ask how often you need to change your pad or tampon on days of heavy bleeding. Not more than every two to three hours is normal.

The first menstrual period

In the past 200 years the age at which a woman has her first period (menarche) has been decreasing. Two hundred years ago, an average woman first menstruated when she was 16^1/$_2$.

A hundred years ago, the average age of first menstruation was 15^1/$_2$. Today an average woman first menstruates when she is between 12^1/$_2$ and 13 years old. 'Average' means that some women menstruate earlier and some later. It is normal for a girl to first menstruate as early as 8 years old or as late as 16.

The downward trend in the age of menarche seems to have levelled in the past thirty years.

Why do women start menstruating earlier today than they did a hundred years ago? Why do ballet dancers first menstruate later than other girls? Why do some athletes stop menstruating when they are in heavy training?

The answers to these questions are not entirely understood. It is thought that until a girl has reached a certain body weight, or probably until the amount of fat in her body reaches a certain proportion of her weight, she will not begin to menstruate. When she reaches this critical level she starts to menstruate, providing that she has secreted enough oestrogen for a number of months to have made her uterus grow to a certain size.

Two hundred years ago, because of frequent illness in childhood and poorer nutrition, girls did not have the critical amount of fat in their bodies to permit menstruation until they were aged 16 or 17. Today, childhood illnesses largely have been eliminated and girls are better nourished, so menarche occurs earlier.

That doesn't explain why ballet dancers start menstruating later, or why female athletes might stop menstruating. Intensive, frequent exercise seems to be the reason. The exercise leads to a decrease in the woman's body fat, and her periods either do not start or cease.

Gymnasts sometimes try to slow puberty not only by exercising but also by restricting their food intake to maintain low body fat, because inadequate nutrition delays skeletal maturation and height.

Gym instructors and ballet teachers are now being counselled to encourage healthy eating (chapter 6) and moderate exercise to assist the normal growth and development of their students.

Feelings about the first period

Many girls do not know very much about what they should expect when they have their first menstrual period.

This is because some mothers do not tell their daughters much, and in many schools sex education (or personal development) lessons do not start until high school. With this lack of knowledge, many young women looking back to their first menstrual period remember that they felt embarrassed, scared, upset, or angry. Other girls had more positive feelings, being excited, happy, or proud when they first menstruated. Before their first period, girls who were able to talk with their mothers, or whose mothers were able to talk to them, felt that they would feel 'grown-up' and be able to have children. However, after menarche many of these girls felt differently.

We asked more than a thousand teenage women what their expectations of menstruation had been before they started menstruating. Half of the young women said that menstruation had been worse than they had expected it would be. Half regarded menstruation as something that happened and that should not be discussed openly, and they did not think they had information to prepare them for menstruation (see table 4.1). In fact, nearly all of the teenage women surveyed would have liked to have known more about menstruation before they reached puberty. Some of their comments included:

- Some mothers are too shy to talk.
- Some mothers hope school will tell us.
- Most information is learnt from friends.
- Some mothers tend to tell their daughters only the basics: 'You're a woman now', meaning just that the young woman can become pregnant.
- Some daughters are embarrassed by the topic.
  Some of the teenage women were quite critical:
- 'My mum gave me all the wrong information. I understood her to say "A bag fills up with blood and bursts when it gets full"—I think she believes this.'
- 'My mother told me nothing, she only told me not to use tampons.'
- 'Mum gave me a book and said I should read it.'
- 'She told me enough not to be terrified at what was happening, but not as much as I know now—and that's not much.'
- 'She explained it was a bleeding at a certain time of the month. It came from an ovarian egg not being fertilised. It might be uncomfortable.'

Table 4.1 Teenage women's experiences of menstruation

Experience	%
Worse than expected	50
Same as expected	7
Better than expected	28
Did not know what to expect	11

On the other hand, some teenage women appreciated what they were told:

- 'They came on my thirteenth birthday. (How lucky!) My mother said it was a gift from God. She was pleased.'
- 'My mother and I can talk about everything. So I asked her questions and she answered them all. I felt good about it when it came.'
- 'She told me about it and that it was natural and there was nothing to hide.'

The ritual of the first period

In our society, menarche is perceived as a private affair, perhaps to be shared with the teenage woman's mother, close friends, but no one else. In some other cultures a woman's first period is a time for ritual or for celebration.

In some societies the young woman is segregated with an older woman to attend her. The young woman has to observe various taboos, which extend to what she may eat and drink. She might be given special tasks or have pain inflicted on her. She might undergo special rituals, which are meant to guarantee her a good sexual response and that she will conceive easily and have a quick and easy childbirth.

In some cultures the period of segregation is also a period of learning, the young woman receiving instruction in sexual and domestic matters from her attendant. In south India in certain cases, a ritual takes place to celebrate the young woman's first period. She sits on a mat of banana leaves, eats raw egg prepared with sugar, and is washed with buffalo milk. When the ceremony is over, the family has a feast, celebrating that the girl is now a mature woman.

Menstrual myths

During a normal menstrual period the blood does not clot, and this was a cause of fear in some cultures: menstrual blood was different from other blood, which always clotted. The people knew that unless bleeding after an injury or a wound was stopped, the person died. They knew that the blood usually clotted and stopped. They also knew that bleeding only followed an accident, an injury, or a wound. But women's menstrual blood came from a hidden place, it didn't clot, it ceased as suddenly as it started, and it recurred at reasonably predictable intervals. No wonder that the people believed that menstrual blood was magical and menstruating women were special.

The magical view of menstrual blood has a long history. Eighteen hundred years ago, Pliny, a woman, wrote a book, *Natural History*, in which she said that if a menstruating woman passed a vineyard, the vines would wither, the grass die, the birds fall, and the wine become sour. Another writer said that if a dog tasted menstrual blood it would go mad. Another wrote that if a man had sexual intercourse with a menstruating woman, he would die, so poisonous was her menstrual flow.

On the other hand, in other societies menstrual blood was thought to have beneficial properties. A woman could bewitch a man if she smeared some menstrual blood on him unawares. In sixteenth-century Europe it was believed that clothes stained with menstrual blood, washed in fresh milk, and hung on a hedge helped an infertile woman to conceive a child.

The peculiar nature of menstrual blood provoked these myths and led to the belief that menstruating women were special and probably dangerous, not only to themselves but also to men. This is the reason why in many societies, as widely different as those of Papua New Guinea and the modern Hindus, menstruating women are either segregated from men or, if living in a family, are restricted in what they may do when menstruating. In rural India, Hindu women may not cook food or work in the fields when menstruating. In Bali, a menstruating woman is not allowed to enter a temple.

Even in Western societies, myths about menstruation persist, and some of these are listed below. Some men (and some women) in Western cultures still believe that menstruation is a symbol of the inferiority of women and that it demonstrates their weaker physical nature. This myth ensures that women only undertake domestic and child-rearing duties. This belief is particularly found in societies in which women talk only to each other about menstruation and where it is thought improper for men to hear about 'women's problems'.

Myths about menstruation

- Women cannot be trusted in important positions because they become irrational in the week before and during menstruation.
- Menstruation cleans the body of dirty blood.
- A woman should douche when menstruation finishes.
- Intercourse should be avoided during menstruation as the man's penis might introduce infection or damage her fragile tissues, and the menstrual blood might damage his penis.
- Menstruation is weakening, so a woman should not play active sports during a period.
- A woman should not get cold or wash her hair during menstruation as the blood might not flow out easily and this could lead to disease.

Why menstrual blood does not clot

Myths about menstruation have a common theme: women's menstrual blood is magical in some way because it does not clot. This, too, is a myth. Menstrual blood, like any other blood, does clot. When it is shed inside the uterus it clots quickly, and then an enzyme in the uterus breaks down the clot so that it becomes, and stays, liquid. This is helpful to women, as the liquid menstrual discharge passes through the cervix more easily than it would if it were in clots. When the blood and tissue lost from the lining of the uterus is excessive, there is not enough of the enzyme to break down all the clots inside the uterus, and the woman might find that she has clots in the menstrual discharge. A few women appear to make tiny clots in the blood when it is in the vagina, but these are not true clots.

They are collections of red blood cells in a meshwork of endometrial tissue.

Attitudes to menstruation

Women have several reasons for wanting to menstruate. In the early 1980s, the World Health Organization asked women in ten countries about their attitudes to menstruation. These countries were Egypt, England, India, Indonesia, Jamaica, Korea, Mexico, Pakistan, the Philippines, and Yugoslavia. In all countries a large number of women, ranging from 45 per cent in England to 95 per cent in Egypt and India, believed that menstruation was necessary for a woman to be a woman—to confirm her femininity. The belief was so strong that, in all the countries, more than half the women (53 per cent in England; 90 per cent in India) would not use a contraceptive that prevented menstruation from occurring. Another reason why many of the women wanted to menstruate regularly was to prove that during the month they had not become pregnant. Rather fewer than half of the women believed that menstruation removed 'waste products' from the body; in other words, it was dirty. Another belief that the women reported was that hair should not be washed during menstruation (more than 60 per cent of Indonesian and Filipino women, to 5 per cent of English women). Another belief held by more than 90 per cent of women, except the English women (54 per cent), was that sexual intercourse should be avoided during menstruation.

When the age of all these women interviewed was checked, 85 per cent were older than 24, and 38 per cent were older than 35. This might have affected the attitudes expressed. By contrast, in a study made in 1984 of adolescent women in Australia, seven out of every ten teenagers considered menstruation a nuisance or an inconvenience (see table 4.2). When asked whether they would prefer not to menstruate if it were safe and reversible, eight out of ten said they would prefer not to.

Thirty per cent of the teenage women said that if they didn't menstruate they would be free of the heaviness and tiredness they felt in the days before their period. On the other hand, many of the women felt that having regular periods indicated that their body was working properly, and a few were reassured that they were not pregnant.

Table 4.2 Teenage Australian women's feelings about menstruation

View of menstruation	%
Inconvenience, nuisance	74
Part of being a woman	13
Doesn't worry me	8
Dirty, disgusting	3
Makes me feel grown up	1
My body is functioning normally	1

As mentioned earlier, in the past many women in many different cultures thought that menstruation was necessary in order to rid the body of toxic substances. If these substances were not able to escape, the woman would become unwell, sick, or sterile. Some of the teenage women surveyed felt that they ought to menstruate 'to get rid of wastes' from their body and that 'the bad blood must get out'. These beliefs are clearly false. Other erroneous beliefs are held by some teenagers—for example, that when menstruating they should avoid getting cold or going out of doors if it was cold and that they should not wash their hair (this was a common belief when their grandmothers were teenagers).

In general, young Australian women have a very practical attitude to menstruation, and only a few hold negative views that menstruation is dirty, revolting, or disgusting. Many young Australian women believe that more information about menstruation should be available and that menstruation should be discussed openly so that myths about menstruation and the belief that it is 'dirty' would be eliminated.

Strange words for menstruation

The mysterious nature of menstrual blood and of menstruation led to the use of a variety of strange euphemisms or slang words to describe menstruation. Instead of calling menstruation a 'period' or a 'menstrual period', many women say that they have 'rags', 'the flowers', 'the curse', 'the visitors', or 'a visit from a friend'. The 'friend' might be given a name—such as George, Henry, Charlie (oddly, most are masculine names). European women more often see menstruation as the 'sickness', the 'monthlies', the 'terms' or the 'courses', 'the time of your grief', or 'them' or 'those'.

These words indicate that menstruation was something very private that should not be talked about openly. It is understandable that women regard menstruation as a private matter, since its absence announces a probable pregnancy and its presence indicates non-pregnancy.

Menstrual protection

By 'menstrual protection' we mean those articles used to absorb menstrual discharge. Until the last sixty years women used rags, which were then thrown away or washed for use in the next menstrual period. In the developed countries most women now use pads or tampons, although some women of certain ethnic groups and women who are environmentally aware continue to use rags.

Almost all women use pads for their first few periods. This is sensible, as it helps a woman to learn about her own patterns of menstrual bleeding. She finds out on what days the heaviest bleeding is likely to occur, how often she has to change her menstrual protection on 'heavy days' and 'light days', and any changes in rate of flow that might appear to occur at night or when exercising. For these reasons, pads offer an advantage over tampons in the first few months or years after menarche, but there is no reason why a woman as young as 12 or 13 should not use tampons, even for her first period. Some young women normally use pads but change to tampons when they want to go swimming.

Some young women still do not know about or are unsure how tampons are used until after they have had their first menstrual period. Some mothers might not tell their daughters about tampons because they find it difficult or embarrassing to explain to their daughters how to use them, or they believe that tampons should not be used until the daughter is older as they have to be inserted into the vagina. Some mothers might also assume that their daughters have learnt about using tampons at school or from magazines. Often teenagers learn about tampons and how to use them from older sisters or friends.

As the teenager grows older she might make the decision to continue using pads, as she finds them comfortable and convenient, or she might decide to change to tampons, because of the convenience that they offer.

Pads

Pads are made from layers of absorbent material inside a layer of polyethylene and a strong, absorbent, perforated paper covering. Pads are made in different thicknesses, shapes, and sizes. The improvement in materials used in the manufacture of pads is constantly reducing their bulkiness but preserving their ability to absorb menstrual fluid, making them acceptable to more women.

Pads are usually described as super, regular, and mini. Most superabsorbent pads can absorb 30–40 mL of fluid, which may contain 25 mL of blood.

The type and size of pad you choose depends on how you feel and the amount of menstrual discharge you have, as the amount you experience varies from month to month, and the day of heaviest bleeding can also vary. Some women feel more secure if they always use the superabsorbent pads, while other women use the superabsorbent pads on days of heavy and intermediate flow and the less absorbent pads when the period is tapering off. There are also panty shields and panty liners, which are even less absorbent than minipads but are used to prevent staining of underpants.

In addition to their usefulness on days of light menstrual flow, minipads can be used when you think your period might be about to start. Minipads can also be used in combination

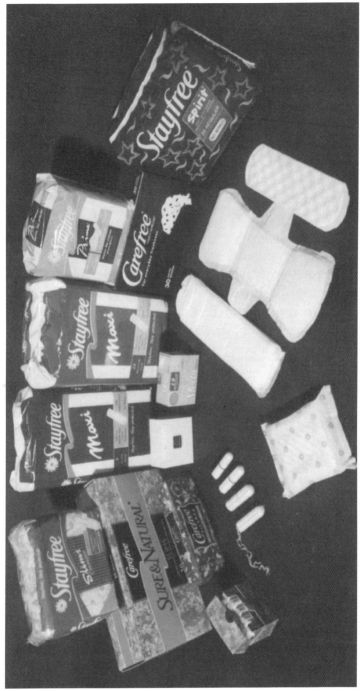

Menstrual protection. Pads and tampons are manufactured in different sizes, shapes, and absorbencies to match different women's needs and lifestyles.

with a tampon on heavier days of bleeding, if you feel the tampon might not be enough to absorb the menstrual discharge and you will be unable to change it in time. Minipads, panty shields, or panty liners can be used for other discharges, such as the watery discharge which occurs when you ovulate. Some women find this discharge can leave a small watermark on light summer clothes.

Most pads have an adhesive strip. A protective strip (which is discarded) is peeled off the back of the pad, which exposes the adhesive on the pad. This adhesive sticks to your underpants and is meant to keep the pad in place.

Some women using pads worry that the pad might show when they wear tight-fitting clothes, such as gym clothes, or that the pad might slip and the menstrual discharge stain their clothes. Other women worry that the blood might run down the side of the pad if they are active. Usually superabsorbent pads hold more menstrual discharge than tampons, but this depends on the brand. For example, some superabsorbent pads hold more than other superabsorbent pads and tampons, while some superabsorbent pads hold only about the same as some superabsorbent tampons. As manufacturers are improving the absorbency of their products, it is worthwhile trying different products every few years to find which are best suited to your needs.

Tampons

Tampons are made of absorbent material like cotton wool, which is tightly compressed. If they are in contact with fluid, they absorb the fluid and expand, like the end of a cotton bud. Like pads they also come in different sizes: super, medium (or regular), and mini. The super tampons can hold as much as 10 mL of fluid, which might contain as much as 6 mL of blood. Different tampons expand in different directions. The tampons that expand sideways are thought to have the advantage of forming a plug, which stops menstrual discharge escaping around the side of the tampon. In fact, as the walls of the vagina fit close to each other, all tampons act as a plug, stopping discharge flowing around the sides of the tampon.

If you place a tampon in a glass of water to see which way it expands when it comes in contact with fluid, do not be alarmed at how big it becomes. When the tampon is inside the vagina it expands only 2–3 mm.

Some women who feel uncomfortable about touching their genitals might feel more relaxed if they use a tampon with an applicator, which can be a double barrel of hard cardboard or plastic, one part sliding inside the other. An applicator gives rigidity when inserting less densely compressed tampons. Most young women prefer to insert a tampon without an applicator; they say that these tampons are easier to insert and more hygienic. Surprisingly, in our study, those women who preferred to use a tampon with an applicator considered that they were easier to insert and the tampon was more hygienic. If you wish to use tampons, choose whichever type you feel most comfortable about using.

For environmental reasons it is best to dispose of tampons in bins or receptacles provided and not flush them down the toilet.

Using a tampon

Many young women find it difficult to insert a tampon on the first few occasions. Some of the teenage women who were surveyed said that they were not sure where 'the hole' is, how hard to push, at what angle to push, or how far to push the tampon in. The instructions provided with the tampons might be difficult to follow. If you become tense and worried, the muscles around the opening to the vagina might also be tense and contract, which makes it even harder to insert the tampon. It is easier to insert a tampon if you are relaxed. There is no 'correct' body position: you can squat, place one leg on a chair or the side of the bath, kneel with legs apart, or lie on the bed with a pillow behind your head and neck. Choose any position in which you feel relaxed, comfortable, and confident.

Confidence is helped by a knowledge of your own body, knowing that you will not accidentally insert the tampon into the 'wrong

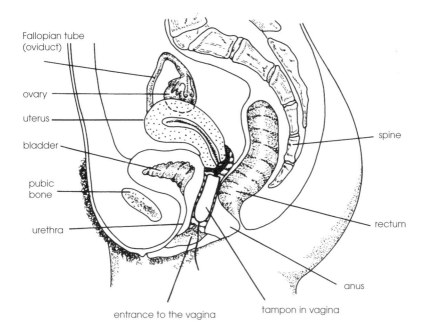

Fallopian tube
(oviduct)

ovary

uterus

bladder

pubic
bone

urethra

spine

rectum

anus

entrance to the vagina

tampon in vagina

Figure 4.1 Where the tampon lies in the vagina.

hole' such as the urethra (the opening to the bladder), that the angle of the vagina is not straight up to your head but upwards and backwards, and that when the tampon is in place in the vagina it cannot be felt at the vaginal entrance. If you can feel a tampon after it is inserted, you need to push it in further, past the muscles that surround the opening to the vagina. You cannot push a tampon in 'too far'; it will not go into the cervix (see figure 4.1).

It is harder to insert a tampon when the vagina is dry. Your vagina might be dry just after you have removed a tampon and on days of light menstrual flow. There are several ways of coping with this. You can push the tampon in a little harder, as you cannot damage the vagina or cervix, or you can wait thirty minutes after removing one tampon before inserting another.

If you choose you can change to a pad or a minipad on days of light flow.

If you find it difficult to insert a tampon on the first few tries and still want to succeed, wait until you do not have your period, coat a tampon liberally with Vaseline (petroleum jelly), and then try. The tampon will slip in easily. Once you know how to do it, you don't need to use Vaseline any more. But you should remember that when you have your period you have to push the tampon in more firmly, as menstrual discharge is not as good a lubricant as Vaseline.

> **Warning** Use only petroleum jelly. Do not use creams, moistur-isers, or oils. They all contain ingredients that can irritate the sensitive tissues of the skin.
>
>   If a tampon is inserted correctly you cannot feel it. If you can feel it, you need to push it a little further into the vagina.

Possible problems

It is possible to forget and leave a tampon in, but not for days or weeks because it will smell. It is also possible to forget that the tampon is still in your vagina and insert another one, but you will usually discover the first one when you try. Even if you don't, your vagina can easily take two tampons. In fact, women who are physically disabled and cannot change tampons or pads every few hours find it extremely helpful to use two at a time.

A tampon can fall out, but only very rarely, usually when you are straining on the toilet. It will not drop out if you are running or exercising as the muscles around the opening to the vagina keep it in.

If you feel you know how to insert a tampon and have tried without success, you may wish to consult your doctor. Tell your doctor your worries and ask for an examination.

Myths

There are many myths about using tampons. The most common myths are listed in the box below. Many women believe that the walls of the vagina are rigid and non-elastic, like the gums in the mouth. In fact the 'tunnel' of the vagina is like your cheeks—if you put large amounts of food in your mouth, the tissue of the

---

Myths about using tampons

- You can't use a tampon until you are 17 because your vagina is too small.
- A tampon is the wrong size and shape for a girl's vagina.
- The hymen has to be 'broken' before you can use a tampon.
- Tampons cause clots in the menstrual discharge and heavy periods.
- You can push a tampon in so far that it will get lost inside you.
- A tampon will damage your vagina or cervix.
- Tampons keep 'bad' blood in your body.
- Tampons cause cancer of the uterus.

---

cheeks can expand. The vagina expands the same way. After all, it stretches to allow a baby to pass through as it is being born.

Many women believe that they lose large volumes of blood, more than 200 mL, at each menstrual period, and they worry if the volume appears to be more or to be less. Because of the difference in the appearance and the size of pads and tampons, some women believe that they are bleeding more, while other women believe they are bleeding less, when using tampons. If women believe they are losing less blood with tampons they might feel their periods are lighter. If they believe that they are bleeding more with tampons they might feel that tampons cause an increase in menstrual flow or that their periods are heavier.

A tampon cannot get lost in your reproductive tract. As figure 4.1 shows, the tampon will always remain in your vagina. Except during childbirth, the opening of the cervix is tiny, no bigger than a drinking straw, so that a tampon couldn't be pushed through it. Oddly, many people believe that during menstruation the reproductive tract opens up. They believe anything that enters the body through the vagina will be able to travel into the rest of the body. As you will realise, this is impossible.

Some women worry that the tampon will damage their hymen. In most young women who are not sexually active, the hymen has a hole in the centre, which is circular or like a half moon, and through which the menstrual discharge passes. If a tampon is inserted it simply stretches this hole, but it is not big enough to break the hymen. As a result, when a woman who uses tampons has sexual intercourse for the first time she might notice some bleeding as the hymen is stretched. This bleeding will not happen if the hymen has been stretched previously, such as by fingers. In a few cases tampons might rupture the hymen—if the hole is not round or semi-lunar but has atypical openings, such as a series of little holes like a sieve, through which the menstrual discharge can pass but a tampon cannot.

Advantages of using tampons
The reasons young women give for deciding to use tampons are: they will not show when you are wearing tight clothes, such as jeans or leotards; you can go swimming and not fear that the blood might show and you cannot feel them when inserted so you can forget you are menstruating.

Many women fear that other people will be able to smell the menstrual discharge on a pad. They cannot, but the woman her-self can and might worry about this, and so chooses to wear tampons as she feels that there is less odour.

The toxic shock syndrome
In 1978, a disease was reported that seemed to be related to the use of tampons. The illness came on suddenly, with high fever, headache, blood-shot eyes, and a bright red rash over the body. In severe cases the woman had vomiting and bad diarrhoea. Her pulse rate rose, and her blood pressure fell. She became cold, and her skin became clammy. In other words, she became 'shocked'. The illness, which was due to a germ called *Staphylococcus aureus*—'the golden staph'—was called toxic shock syndrome (TSS). Although TSS can occur during tampon use, it can occur in non-tampon users.

Toxic shock is unusual, and the chance of getting it from the use of tampons is less than one in 40,000. If you use the pre-cautions mentioned below, toxic shock is very unlikely to occur. Before inserting the tampon you should wash your hands.

However, there is no hygienic or medical advantage in using a tampon enclosed in an applicator: its use is a matter of personal choice.

- The tampon should be changed when necessary but should not be left in the vagina for longer than eight hours before being replaced.
- At night you should not use a tampon. Instead you should choose a pad or a minipad, depending on the volume of your menstrual discharge.
- If you develop fever (higher than 38.9 degrees Celsius), headache, dizziness, aching muscles, and occasionally vomiting or diarrhoea during menstruation, remove the tampon and consult your doctor.

Menstrual problems

Premenstrual problems

Many teenagers know, two or three days in advance, that they are about to menstruate. They complain that their 'stomach is swollen', or they develop a headache or have dark rings beneath their eyes. About one teenage woman in every three complains of feeling irritable or tired during the days just before, or the first days of, menstruation. These symptoms are normal, although disturbing. If these symptoms are distressing keep a daily diary (to make sure they are always premenstrual) and take the diary with you to your doctor. Exercise, 'normal eating' (see chapter 6), and relaxation should be tried before medications are used. The pill can help the symptoms or make them worse.

Painful crampy periods

Some time during the two years following the onset of menstruation, nearly three-quarters of young women will develop crampy pains that start a few hours before menstruation and might last for the first one or two days of menstruation.

The crampy menstruation pains have been given the medical name of dysmenorrhoea. The discomfort is mild in nearly half of the women who have dysmenorrhoea. It does not affect the woman's activities, although she feels some discomfort in her pelvis.

Nearly one woman in three has more severe dysmenorrhoea that affects her activities to some degree, and about one woman in five has severe dysmenorrhoea that is incapacitating (see table 4.3). Women who have dysmenorrhoea as severely as this usually have to go to bed and lie quietly for about twelve hours. Typically the crampy pains are felt in the lower abdomen, but they might radiate into the back and down the legs. Half of the young women who have severe dysmenorrhoea also have other uncomfortable symptoms, including nausea, vomiting, diarrhoea, headache, dizziness, and nervousness.

The severity of the menstrual cramps can vary from month to month. Some teenagers have 'bad' months most of the time, others have only occasional 'bad' months. Menstrual cramps cause pain. They might lead to absence from work or from school. If they occur during a school examination they might disadvantage the woman. If they occur when she has a sporting or social engagement they might prevent her from participating

Table 4.3   Proportion of young women affected by crampy periods

Experience	%
Menstruation not painful	28
Daily activities not affected	
Menstruation mildly painful	34
Analgesics not often needed	
Menstruation painful	23
Daily activities affected	
Analgesics give relief	
Menstruation very painful: often headaches, tiredness, vomiting, diarrhoea	15
Daily activities severely affected	
Analgesics poor effect; anti-prostaglandin drug usually effective	

in a pleasurable activity. They lead to many visits to a doctor by teenage women aged between 16 and 19. One survey found that 8 per cent of teenage women had visited a doctor in the previous twelve months because of dysmenorrhoea. In Sweden, a survey of 19-year-old women living in Gothenburg showed that 21 per cent attended a doctor because of menstrual cramps. They usually affect women younger than 25, and for some reason tend to disappear, or become less severe, after that time.

The cause of menstrual cramps has been found. They are due to substances called prostaglandins. Prostaglandins are made in many organs of the body, and there are several kinds of prostaglandin. The particular prostaglandins involved in dysmenorrhoea are called PGE2 and PGF2-alpha. The quantity of these prostaglandins increases as menstruation approaches, provided that the woman has ovulated. When ovulation occurs, the female sex hormone progesterone is made in the ovary. Progesterone alters the character of the lining of the uterus, making it soft and fleshy. Progesterone also induces the cells that make up the lining to manufacture (synthesise) PGF2-alpha. This occurs in every woman who ovulates, but in women who have dysmenorrhoea, more PGF2-alpha seeps from the lining of the uterus into its muscle where it acts on the muscle cells, making them go into a cramp or spasm. It also makes the muscles in the walls of the blood vessels supplying the muscles go into spasm, with the result that the cramps become more severe.

The reason why some teenage women produce more PGF2-alpha than others is not understood, but it might be familial. It has been found that daughters react to menstrual cramps in a way similar to their mothers. If the mother did not have dysmenorrhoea, only 6 per cent of daughters regularly complained of dysmenorrhoea, but if the mother had dysmenorrhoea when she was young, 30 per cent of their daughters suffered regularly from dysmenorrhoea.

For many years aspirin or paracetamol have been a treatment given by mothers to their daughters for menstrual cramps. In mild cases aspirin worked very well. Now that it is known that excessive PGF2-alpha in the uterus is the cause of dysmenorrhoea, we know why aspirin worked well. Aspirin reduces the production of prostaglandin. Unfortunately to reduce it completely would require such a large dose of aspirin that it could cause dangerous side effects, such as stomach bleeding.

New products, given the name of non-steroidal anti-inflammatory drugs (NSAIDS), have been made, which are more effective than aspirin in treating menstrual cramps. These drugs not only reduce the synthesis of PGF2-alpha but also stop it from binding to the muscle cells. Several anti-prostaglandin drugs are available, and none seems more effective than any other. But if one does not work, or causes side effects, another may be tried. Most doctors start by giving mefenamic acid (Ponstan), and if

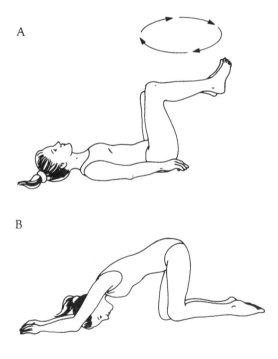

Figure 4.2 Some exercises to help relieve menstrual cramps. (a) Lie on your back with your knees up and together. Describe a small circle in the air with your knees. (b) Kneel on the floor, and place your forehead on the ground between your elbows. In this position your uterus is hanging down, which helps it to relax.

it fails to relieve the cramps, they choose naproxen (Naprosyn), flufenamic acid (Arlef), ibuprofen (Brufen), or diclofenac (Voltarin). The medication is taken either when the cramps begin or, if other symptoms start before the cramps, when these other symptoms begin. The medications should be taken with food as they might cause some 'tummy upsets'—bloating, nausea, or discomfort. A woman who takes these drugs might find that her menstrual period is shorter and the amount of menstrual discharge less. The antiprostaglandin drugs relieve severe menstrual cramps in more than 80 per cent of women.

There is an alternative treatment, which is for the young woman to take a contraceptive pill. The pill works by suppressing ovulation. Since the woman does not ovulate, progesterone is not released by the ovary, which reduces the amount of PGF2-alpha in the uterus.

Some women, however, choose not to take drugs to relieve menstrual cramps, for a variety of reasons. If this is the case, the woman may relieve painful cramps by doing the exercises described in figure 4.2, or by lying down and placing a hot water bag on her abdomen.

Teenage women and doctors

Many teenage women find that they need to visit a doctor about a gynaecological (woman's) problem. A common reason for visiting a doctor is that the young woman has problems with her periods, which might be painful, too heavy, or occurring too often or too infrequently. Another reason is that the teenager is worried about a vaginal discharge or because she wants to learn more about contraception.

The first contact with the doctor is important. If the doctor does not make the teenager feel comfortable, the visit might be ineffective. If the teenager is reluctant to answer the questions the doctor will ask, the visit might be fruitless.

The kind of question the doctor will ask will depend on the teenager's problem. For example, if the visit is because of a problem about menstruation, she will probably be asked some of the following questions:

- How old were you when you had your first period?
- How often do your periods occur, that is, how many days are there between the first day of one period and the first day of the next period?
- For how many days do you menstruate?
- Do you have any pains (cramps) with your period?
- Do you have any problems in the week before your period starts?
- How often do you change your pad or tampon on days of heavy bleeding?
- Is the pad or tampon soaked through when you change it?
- Do you have any 'break-through' bleeding or spotting between your periods?
- Do you know if your mother or older sister had any problems with their periods?
- Are there any other questions about menstruation that you would like to ask?

Sometimes the doctor will suggest that the teenager needs to be examined internally; in other words, the doctor performs a pelvic examination. If you have never been examined in this way, the idea might be frightening. So that you don't become too anxious, let us describe what the doctor does.

First, the doctor will ask you to empty your bladder, then to undress from your waist down and lie comfortably on a couch, so that your abdomen can be examined. You may lie under a sheet, or not, as you prefer. It depends on your feelings. After looking at your abdomen, your doctor will gently press one hand over its various parts to find out whether you have any lumps or tender areas.

Next your doctor will ask you to draw up your legs and let your knees fall apart, so that your external genitals can be examined. Because of the cultural significance of the hymen, if you are a virgin your doctor will probably not examine your vagina. If you have had sex your doctor might ask permission to introduce a speculum into your vagina. A speculum is a

A

B

C

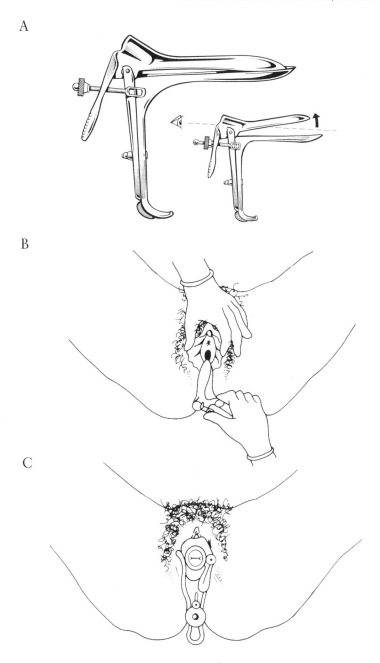

Figure 4.3 A speculum examination. (a) A speculum. (b) Inserting the speculum. (c) Speculum open in vagina to expose the cervix.

small metal or plastic instrument that enables the doctor to look at the vaginal walls and the cervix (see figure 4.3). If the teenager has a vaginal discharge, using a speculum enables the doctor to take a swab from the upper part of the vagina, which is then sent to a laboratory to identify the cause of the discharge. If the speculum is warm and moist, and is introduced gently, it is generally not painful, although it might be a little uncomfortable. The more you can relax, the less discomfort you will experience.

Once the doctor has inspected your vagina and cervix, the speculum is removed. The doctor will now want to examine you to feel the size and shape of your uterus and to find out whether your Fallopian tubes are swollen or painful. To do this the doctor inserts one or two fingers into your vagina and places the other hand on your abdomen. This helps the doctor to feel your uterus and Fallopian tubes between the fingers of both hands. Again, this is usually not uncomfortable, provided the doctor is gentle and you are able to relax. If you have not had sexual intercourse, the doctor will omit the speculum and vaginal examination, but to find out more about your genital organs, the doctor might suggest that you make an appointment to have a pelvic ultrasound (sound picture). This is a bit like having a computer mouse moved over your abdomen. While this is happening the radiographer will show you the picture of your organs on a computer screen. After the examination the doctor will leave you while you put on your clothes. Then you have the opportunity of talking with your doctor, who will explain any findings to you and talk about your problem.

If you are sexually active, your doctor might suggest that you have a Pap smear. This is a test to find out whether you have cancer of your cervix (or abnormal cells that might lead to cancer). The test is called a Pap smear because it was introduced by Dr Papanicolaou, an American gynaecologist, more than forty years ago. The smear is made by exposing the cervix by means of a vaginal speculum during a pelvic examination. Some of the cells that cover the cervix are scraped off gently by a soft plastic brush (see figure 4.4). The doctor then smears the cells on to a microscope slide and sends the slide to a laboratory, where it is stained and examined.

It is recommended that any sexually active woman should have a Pap smear taken every two years, commencing within two years of first being sexually active up until 70 years of age This is because it is thought that one of the things that might cause cancer of the cervix is a virus, the wart virus, which is passed between people during sexual intercourse. If any abnormalities are found, more frequent Pap smears are recommended.

Nowdays there are Pap test registers which remind women if their routine Pap smear is three months overdue. Your doctor will discuss this with you.

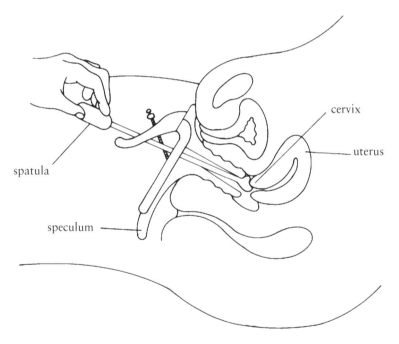

Figure 4.4 Taking a Pap smear.

Chapter Five

Adolescent behaviour

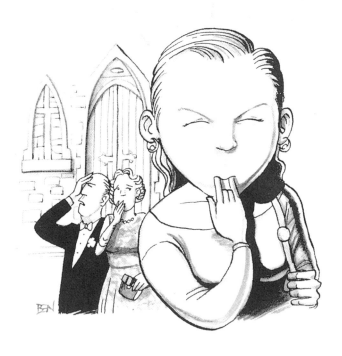

Why be disagreeable when with a little help
you can be impossible?

Arthur Murphy

Many adults believe that teenagers reject all the beliefs of their parents. They believe that teenagers are disobedient, disrespectful, untidy, and often physically dirty, and that these attitudes cause a 'generation gap' between teenagers and their parents.

Of course many teenagers have ideas and attitudes that differ from those of their parents, just as their parents disagreed with their own parents when they were teenagers. It is not surprising that teenagers sometimes argue with their parents, disagree with them, and disobey them. Of course some teenagers are criticised by their parents for the way they dress and the way they do their hair. Teenagers do have swings of moods from black despair to high elation. They are often untidy, occasionally lazy, and sometimes noisy. Such behaviour is normal in adolescence, and it is likely that parents of today behaved in a similar way when they were teenagers.

In the fifth century BC Socrates complained: 'Our youth now love luxury. They have bad manners, contempt for authority. They show disrespect for elders and love chatter in place of exercise . . . They contradict their parents, chatter before company, gobble up their food, and tyrannise their teachers.'

Attaining independence

Adolescence is a period of transition, when teenagers move from total dependence on their parents to relative independence. During the transition the young woman is growing up and discovering that she is a unique person and should be respected for that. Adolescence is also a time when the teenager must learn how to interact independently with other people and understand how society expects her to behave. During this time the teenager learns to work out for herself the right way to behave, rather than simply doing as she is told. This might cause conflict and irritation between parents and teenagers, but there is no unbridgeable 'generation gap', although this term is often used to explain why some parents and children fail to agree on certain issues.

In fact, most teenagers want to please their parents. Most teenagers admire and respect their parents (although they argue with them), and agree with them on most important matters. Rather than a widening generation gap, in recent years parents and their daughters seem to have been drawn together.

Some teenagers and their parents have problems: some teenagers rebel or withdraw; some become perverse. On the other hand, some parents are unnecessarily strict, cruel, brutal, or indifferent to their daughters' needs. But these problem teenagers and problem parents are a minority. Most relationships between teenagers and their parents are good. Most parents and teenagers can talk *with* each other (not *at* each other), and most teenagers turn to their parents for guidance on many major concerns. In minor things they might disagree. One English study found that nearly half of the parents disapproved of their daughter's hairstyle or clothes, and nearly a third had arguments about the time their 16-year-old daughter came home or went to bed. But on major domestic concerns there was general agreement. Only 7 per cent of parents had major disagreements with their daughter as often as once a month, and half of those who did had them once per week or more often.

Some parents believe that these days teenage daughters behave very differently to the way *they* behaved as teenagers. They believe that the world is very different now and much more dangerous. There are many more drugs available; more teenagers are sexually active; sexually transmitted diseases, including HIV–AIDS, are more common; and more teenagers have cars and drive them dangerously. Looking back on their time as teenagers, today's parents believe that they had set rules and defined boundaries, and that if they did not obey the rules they were punished. When they were teenagers they only listened to loud music; sexually they felt they had behaved responsibly; they went out less often; and they obeyed their parents more than their daughters obey them. They wonder whether their adolescent daughters have been disadvantaged and exposed to danger because they have relaxed the rules and have not set the boundaries their parents set for them.

It is true that the media are more pervasive than twenty-five years ago: advertising is more relentless, soapies are directed at teenagers, explicit videos and video games are available and uncensored material is accessible on the Internet; all of which might influence teenagers' behaviour. But people's memories are fickle and selective. It is probable that today's parents were perceived as 'wild' by their parents just as they perceive their daughters today.

This is not to say that parents should not set limits on teenagers' activities. They should, or their teenage daughters will become anxious. The limits should not be rigid, but flexible and adjusted as the teenager matures and becomes more capable of handling her life. David Bennett, head of the Adolescent Unit at the Children's Hospital in Sydney, writes in his book *Growing Pains*: 'If limits are not clearly set, children (and teenagers) feel distinctly insecure and will come to interpret it as a lack of caring.'

Adolescence is a time for a person to discover who she is, for her to feel good about herself, and to develop self-esteem. It is a time when the teenager is torn between the wish to define her own personality—to be herself—and, at the same time, the need to 'belong'. Some teenagers find the process difficult, becoming miserable and anxious about themselves, but most come through the experience happily.

During the adolescent years, the teenager has a number of specific needs and wants. The fulfilment of these needs and wants (listed below) enables the teenager to develop into an assured and well-balanced adult.

- Teenagers need social acceptance, to be welcomed into a special group.
- Teenagers seek social acceptance, that is, achievement within the group.
- Teenagers need friendship and intimacy.
- Teenagers seek their own identity.
- Teenagers need their own 'space'.
- Teenagers seek independence.
- Teenagers need some degree of conformity, but with their peers rather than their parents.

- Teenagers also need to know that their parents love them and that the limits they set are not arbitrary.

When you are a child, most of your friendships occur because you and your friends like doing the same activities. When you become a teenager, your friendships involve a much deeper relationship. You want to share your deeper feelings, you want to exchange ideas, you want to feel comfortable and to be able to disclose intimate matters to each other. This might lead you to join a group or, more usually, to have a special friend. The members of the group change often and might be made up of the same or of both sexes. Special friends change too, one special friend being replaced by another after a period of emotional unhappiness. In the earlier teenage years the special friend is usually female; in the later teenage years the special friend can be male. This means that adolescence is a period in which you accept the influence of your friends (called your 'peer group') more readily, and their influence on your behaviour becomes increasingly strong while that of your parents declines.

The need for intimacy with the special friend is expressed by wanting to spend most of the time with her or him: by long telephone calls (to the annoyance of some parents), and by 'hanging about' together, often doing nothing more than being together. Special girlfriends tend to be of similar ages but, in later relationships with males, the man tends to be older. As the relationship develops, the teenager spends increasing amounts of time with her 'special friend' and less time with her family. However, most teenagers still enjoy the time they spend with their families.

Parents and daughters

Several studies about what daughters think of their parents and what parents think of their daughters have been made, mainly in the USA. They show some of the ways each side thinks of the other. First, teenage daughters made these comments about their parents:

- 'My parents always complain and tell me what to do.'
- 'They never see my point of view. They give me the "When I was young" speech.'
- 'Mum worries about my dates and doesn't trust me.'
- 'They are too overprotective and anxious that something bad is going to happen to me.'
- 'My parents are too concerned about my school grades.'
- 'They are always on about coming home late.'

Second, parents (usually the mother) made these comments about their daughters:

- 'She wants everything now and feels she deserves everything.'
- 'She keeps trying to push me to my limit.'
- 'She doesn't understand that parents have problems too.'
- 'She needs a "curfew" so that she learns responsibility.'
- 'She is always on the phone; her room is always untidy.'

In spite of these comments (which are extremes), most parents and their daughters relate well, but some need to ask: how can we improve our relationship? Do we always blame each other for our problem? Do we make enough time to talk with each other?

If a problem does arise it is better for parents to negotiate, to discuss the problem, rather than just give orders. Some parents have to realise that their daughter is growing up and they have to begin to let go, allowing her some independence, hard though this might be.

Here is a message for parents. There is not much point in trying to negotiate in the middle of a fight. There is no point in screaming at your teenage daughter no matter how much you might want to, because she won't listen. Walk away and, when the anger of both of you has calmed, try to talk with her. It might help for both of you to go out of the house, with all its memories of the fight, to do this successfully.

Who am I?

'We cannot know ourselves, be intimate with others, until we know who we are, until we have found our identity.' The teenage years are a time when the person is trying to find an answer to the question: who am I? It is not an easy question to answer, but a teenager has a better chance than a child of answering it because, with increasing maturity, she has developed the capacity for abstract thought. For example, a child shown pictures of a cherry, a tomato, and a plum might say: 'You can eat them' or 'They are all red', but a teenager might add to this: 'They are all examples of fruit.' This is a simple example of abstract thought.

Abstract thought is needed to answer the question: who am I? The actual question is rarely asked, but the answer to it underlies a substantial part of a teenager's thoughts and considerably influences a teenager's behaviour.

The subconscious need to know who you are can be explored during the teenage years in several ways, and different teenagers choose different roads. One important way of exploring the question is fantasy. Fantasy and day-dreaming are important to most teenagers. Through fantasy a person can test responses to other people and to new situations. In a young woman's fantasy world she is always successful, always popular, beautiful, powerful, and independent. Fantasy can be increased by reading or by watching TV. Reading, particularly, projects the reader into an imaginary fantastic world and increases the imagination. TV is less effective, as the viewer is provided with a complete scenario, so that your imagination is less stimulated. But TV is more pervasive and influential than reading, as TV is watched for thirty hours a week by average teenagers, whereas most teenagers read for fewer than four hours each week.

The question 'Who am I?' is also explored by involvement with others, by identifying with a rock star, or a TV soapie star, or a sporting hero, however briefly. The hidden question is: 'Am I like her—could she be me?' The teenager temporarily identifies with the heroine, moving on when she finds that the identification doesn't work.

An answer to the question 'Who am I?' is also sought by joining and conforming to the behaviour of a group. This might mean that the teenager wears bizarre clothes, has weird hairstyles, and behaves in a way her parents find disturbing. Usually the trend passes, and the young woman finds another group with which to identify or becomes more involved in a relationship with one person.

The question 'Who am I?' causes a teenager to be concerned about how other people feel about her. In childhood, for example, a girl might say: 'I hate my teacher'. In adolescence she is more likely to say: 'My teacher hates me'. Thus, the teenage woman has become less self-centred and more concerned about how others perceive her.

Most teenagers have 'secret lives'. There are some thoughts that teenagers want to keep secret from their parents. There are some things teenagers do that they don't want their parents to know about. The extent of a teenager's 'secret life' depends largely on the degree of her parents' secrecy. Most parents do

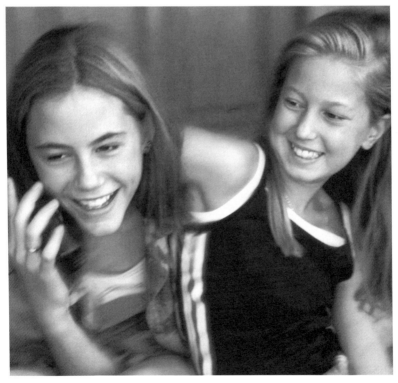

During adolescence teenagers spend increasing amounts of time with their friends. The need to belong is strong.

not tell their children their secrets, and the more they can be open with their teenage children, the less the teenager will keep secrets from them.

Many teenagers have worries that they keep to themselves or that they reveal to their family and friends. The following concerns were expressed by Canadian teenagers in a survey:

- What will my future be? Will I get a job?
- Am I attractive to others?
- Should I have, and enjoy, sexual feelings?
- Do other people like me?
- How can I get along with my parents?

Eventually most teenagers are able to answer the question: 'Who am I?' Some fail. Those who succeed best in finding their identity feel good about themselves, relate well with others, avoid being dominated by others, and master some tasks they perceive as important.

As well as searching for an identity, a teenager seeks to become increasingly independent. In our society a male teenager is pushed more strongly towards independence than a female teenager. A young woman is often still expected to remain dependent on her parents for longer and later on her husband, at least while they have children, although this expectation has decreased in recent years.

The search for independence means that a teenage woman might behave in ways that cause anxiety to her parents. She begins to question some of their values. She expects to have a 'space' of her own. In mid adolescence this is often her room, which, in her parents' opinion, has become a mess. The bed is unmade, the room is strewn with clothes, books, computer games, and CDs. If she is forced to tidy it up she is resentful, and the room rapidly resumes its chaotic state. The messiness of her 'space' might be complemented by a messiness of herself, at least as seen by others. As the girl grows older, the messiness often changes to a meticulous neatness or to the adoption of the 'uniform' of her chosen group.

The achievement of independence is aided if the parents are neither overstrict nor overpermissive.

School

School also helps the discovery of 'Who am I?' School provides interaction with peers with differing cultural, political, and religious beliefs, and a range of interests and activities. Many schools are trying to improve the 'self-esteem' of young women by:

- Providing a safe, protective environment, and promoting the value of differences between people.
- Supporting enjoyable groups that make teenagers feel better about themselves.
- Supporting a wide range of activities to allow all teenagers to find out what they are good at and enjoy.
- Encouraging peer support by older students.
- Not supporting physical or mental bullying, 'bitchiness', or isolation of students by other students.
- Training teachers not to inadvertently undermine a student's self-esteem or humiliate her.
- Supporting early referral to school counsellors and health professionals of students perceived as not coping as well as usual.

If you are feeling unhappy and rejected at school, it is important to talk to someone: an older sister, a trusted teacher, a parent, or school counsellor are all people you can talk with. You do not deserve to be made to feel this way. It will get better. Help must be sought for any bullying as soon as it occurs.

Early and late maturers

Most girls reach menarche—start to menstruate—between the ages of $12^{1}/_{2}$ and $13^{1}/_{2}$. A few start earlier and some start later. The reason for this difference is not clear, although we have mentioned that excessive exercise or strict dieting (because of a fear of becoming fat) could delay the onset of menarche.

The effect of starting to menstruate earlier, or of having a delayed menarche, on a girl's feelings and behaviour is not clear. Some 'early maturers' seem to be better able to adjust and are more popular and more confident than some late maturers, but in other cases no differences have been found. A possible explanation is that the later maturer feels inferior to her friends and has less self-esteem because all her friends have begun menstruating, because her breasts are small or non-existent, and because she has fewer sexual feelings than her friends. Sexuality and sexual feelings are important to teenagers, and they talk a lot about the subject. However, earlier maturers might have problems. Early maturers have sexual feelings and explore their sexuality at an earlier age. For this reason they are more likely to have an unwelcome pregnancy during their early teenage years.

Chapter Six

Eating well

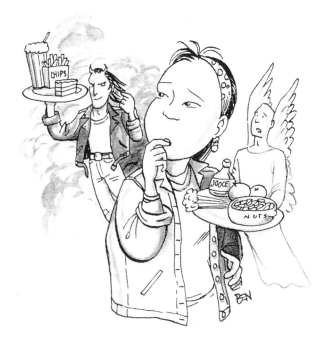

Fast food: they should flush it down the toilet
and cut out the middle man.

Ben Elton

Most parents want their children to be healthy and to look well fed. Most parents are happy when their children eat everything that is put in front of them and unhappy when they reject food. Most young children eat what their parents give them or tell their parents their food likes and dislikes.

In the teenage years this pattern changes. Teenagers tend to eat away from home with their friends more often than they did as children, although for many the evening meal at home is still the largest meal of the day. Eating out at 'fast food' places, or snacking, is enjoyable, and it gives the individual a feeling of independence—of finding their own identity.

As well as this, teenagers tend to develop certain food habits (see table 6.1). About one teenager in five (usually female) misses eating breakfast. But teenagers make up for this by snacking or eating sweets. In the United States this behaviour is called 'grazing'. It means that the teenager goes into a shop or a fast food outlet on impulse and buys a snack. Most teenagers 'graze' at least once a day, and they might buy snack foods twice a day or more often. Most snack foods contain more fat, sugar, and salt than is good for you if you eat a lot of them, but they taste good and are 'fun' foods. As well as eating chocolate bars, lollies, cakes, potato chips, and similar snack foods, many

Table 6.1 Teenagers' food likes and dislikes

Likes	Dislikes
Hamburgers	Liver
French fries	Salads
Ice cream	Fish (other than fried in batter)
Take-away fried chicken	Cabbage
Pizzas	Spinach
Milk shakes	Casseroles
Coca Cola or Pepsi	Spaghetti
Hot dogs	
Lollies, sweets	
Chocolate bars	

teenagers eat fast foods such as hamburgers, fried chicken, pizza, and fish and chips. These fast foods are more nutritionally balanced than the other snack foods, and fast food outlets have a good deal to offer teenagers. The food is relatively cheap. The place is enjoyable: you can eat as slowly or as quickly as you want, and you meet a lot of other teenagers and have fun.

Eating satisfies our energy requirements. Because of their high growth rate, teenagers need extra energy, and they generally enjoy eating. Most teenagers get enough to eat and often more than enough. If you eat more than you need to meet your daily expenditure of energy, you will slowly but surely become overweight and eventually obese. By late adolescence about 10 per cent of teenagers are obese. As well, if you eat large amounts of food that is not particularly nutritious, you might develop health problems later in life. Most people do not choose food because it is nutritious. They choose foods because it tastes good, it is familiar to the eater, it looks good, and it helps people to socialise. This means that different age groups often choose different foods. Teenagers enjoy snacks, hamburgers and chips, soft drinks, fast foods, chocolate, and lollies.

Changes in dietary habits

It is only in the past fifty years or so that teenagers have been able to buy these snack foods in any quantity, and over this time the eating behaviour of most people living in the rich industrialised countries has changed. In this time a much wider choice of foods has become available, and more people are eating at fast food places or buying take-away foods. Restaurants and take-away food shops providing Chinese, Thai, Indian, and Japanese foods are becoming increasingly common. These, in addition to pizza, pasta, and hamburger outlets, provide a wide range of food choices.

As well as changes in what teenagers eat, changes have occurred in what people of all ages eat. A hundred and fifty years ago, most people's daily diet consisted largely of grain-based foods (wheat, rice, barley, corn, and oats) and vegetables, particularly potatoes and greens, and only a small amount of meat. Fruits and vegetables were eaten when in season.

Today, the proportion of unrefined carbohydrates and whole grains (i.e., obtained from breads, cereals, legumes, fruit and vegetables) in the daily diets of many people living in the rich countries of the world has fallen. At the same time, more meat and prepared foods, such as pastries, cakes, biscuits, confectionery, and take-away foods, which contain 'hidden' fat, sugar, and salt, are being eaten. Soft drinks are being increasingly consumed. These changes have increased the amount of fat, particularly saturated (i.e., animal) fat, and sugar, and have halved the quantity of dietary fibre that we eat each day.

Most people enjoy eating foods that are rich in fats. Fats include saturated fat, which is involved in the development of heart disease, mono-unsaturated fats, and polyunsaturated fats. Most foods that contain fat have a proportion of each of these types of fat, but some have a good deal of saturated fat. Sometimes the fat is obvious. If you buy butter or margarine at the supermarket, you know that you are buying fat. If you buy beef or lamb with an outer layer of fat, you can see the fat. But fat is also cleverly 'hidden' in potato chips, croissants, cheese, cakes, biscuits, sauces, and in many take-away foods. It is these saturated fats that are 'harmful' if eaten in large amounts as they, along with smoking and lack of exercise, increase the risk of heart disease.

Fats in food are not all bad. Fats have several advantages: they improve the taste of foods and carry flavour; they provide a concentrated source of energy; and they provide vitamins A and D, which are fat-soluble and are needed to keep us healthy. Some fats are known as essential fatty acids (omega-3 and omega-6 fatty acids); your body cannot produce them and they are essential for good health. These are called polyunsaturated fats and are in oily fish, nuts, and certain cooking oils.

Our diet today contains less dietary fibre than the diet of our great-great-grandparents. The amount of dietary fibre that we eat has diminished because we no longer eat as much whole grain breads and cereals, legumes, fruits, and vegetables, which are good sources of dietary fibre.

'Western lifestyle' diseases

Most nutritionists believe that these changes in diet—more sugar, fat, and salt, and less fibre combined with less exercise—are the main cause of the increasing prevalence of 'Western lifestyle' diseases over the last 150 years. These diseases are:

- coronary heart disease
- high blood pressure
- obesity
- some bowel diseases
- adult onset diabetes
- dental disease
- osteoporosis.

The diseases (with the exception of dental diseases) are more likely to affect middle-aged or elderly people, but there is increasing evidence that children and teenagers are starting to suffer from these diseases and, in addition, what you eat when you are a teenager could affect your health in later life.

Coronary heart disease

Scientists agree that if a person habitually eats food that contains a lot of saturated fat, not only is the person likely to become fat but also the level of cholesterol in her or his blood may rise. High blood cholesterol is one of the risk factors for coronary heart disease. (Other risk factors are smoking, lack of exercise, diabetes, and obesity.) In the past century, the number of people aged between 40 and 70 who have had a heart attack has been increasing, and has levelled off only in the past twenty years. This is due to the fact that many people in Western countries have become aware of the risk factors of heart disease and have reduced the amount of saturated fats in their diets, are exercising more, and have stopped smoking.

High blood pressure

Many obese people have high blood pressure. This increases their chance of having a stroke or a heart attack. Many nutritionists think that if people eat too much salt, they are more likely to develop high blood pressure.

Obesity

The greater range of good-tasting foods that are readily available from many outlets means that people eat not because they are hungry, but because they enjoy eating, because it is a social activity. Foods high in fat, while they taste good, do not help you to feel 'full', so most people eat more of them than they need. If, over the years, you regularly take more energy into your body than you use, you will slowly but inevitably gain weight. Most people do not want to gain weight, which is the reason for the many weight clinics found in towns and cities and the slimming diets published frequently in books and magazines. However, many people find it hard or impossible to keep to the diets, and any weight they lose tends to return.

Hard as people might try to watch their weight, the number of overweight and obese people in Western societies is increasing. By the age of 50, 18 per cent of women in Australia will be obese. Obesity increases a person's chances of developing some other illnesses, including high blood pressure, gallstones, and diabetes.

Bowel diseases

The increase of animal fat in the diet together with the decrease in the amount of dietary fibre eaten is the most likely cause of a number of bowel diseases common among people who eat a Western diet and live a Western lifestyle (the diseases are much less common in developing countries). These diseases include constipation, haemorrhoids, appendicitis, 'irritable bowel', and bowel cancer.

Diabetes

Type 2 diabetes, adult onset diabetes or non-insulin-dependent diabetes is being diagnosed increasingly among women and men in their forties. One cause of this increase is believed to be too much energy in our diet, in the form of fat, combined with too little exercise. If we eat foods containing less fat and aim to do more daily physical activity we will be less likely to become obese and develop type 2 diabetes.

Dental disease

Your teeth are mainly made up of a tough bone called dentine, over which there is a thin coat of enamel (this is the hardest tissue in the body). Inside the dentine is the tooth pulp, which contains nerves and blood vessels. When food containing particles of sugar sticks in the crevices between the teeth, or on the surface of the teeth, it interacts with the saliva and the myriad bacteria that are always in the mouth. This interaction forms a substance called plaque. The plaque sticks to the surface of the tooth, and one of the bacteria converts glucose in the food into a substance called destran. The destran is used by another type of bacteria (*lactobacilli*) for growth. Some of it is turned into an acid. The acid in the plaque gradually eats into the dentine through cracks in the tooth enamel, and dental caries start.

Until about thirty years ago, a large number of teenagers had dental disease, usually dental caries, an average of five teeth having decayed by the age of 18. One of the causes of dental caries was the amount of sugar-rich foods and soft drinks consumed by the teenagers. Today, far fewer teenagers have dental decay, because teenagers' teeth have improved because fluoride is added to the water supply. Fluoride hardens the tooth enamel and prevents cracks forming, so that acid cannot reach the dentine.

Fluoride also helps the dentine to heal so that, even if acid gets into the dentine, it has less chance of forming a decayed area.

However, fluoridation of the water supply is not enough to avoid dental disease. Dental caries can be reduced further if people clean their teeth regularly and if they avoid drinking sweetened soft drinks and eating sugary snacks (as far as possible), if they have snack foods, such as dairy products and fruit that are protective to teeth, and visit their dentist regularly.

Osteoporosis

As more women are living longer, a bone condition called osteoporosis has become more common. In osteoporosis, the bones of the spine, the thigh bones, and the wrist bones become brittle. If the woman does not take action to prevent osteoporosis, some of the vertebrae of her spine might collapse. She becomes shorter, her back becomes bent, and a hump develops in the upper part of her spine. She might also develop severe backache. If she trips and falls, she could break her leg or her wrist.

Osteoporosis is largely preventable, at least until old age. If you have strong bones you are less likely to develop osteoporosis. Calcium makes your bones strong, but only when they are gaining strength. By the time you are 30 years of age your bones are as strong as they ever will be. This means that young women should

Table 6.2 Best sources of calcium (you need 1000 mg per day)

Source	Portion	Calcium
Milk	1 cup	310 mg
Cheese	40g	310 mg
Yoghurt	1 tub (200 gm)	250 mg
Custard	1/4 cup (125 ml)	140 mg
Fortified soy milk	1 cup	300 mg
Canned salmon with bones	1/2 cup	280 mg
Tinned sardines	5	285 mg
Evaporated milk	1 cup	650 mg
Broccoli	1 cup	98 mg

try to make their bones as strong as possible by eating a diet that provides at least 1000 mg of calcium each day and by exercising regularly. The best sources of calcium are shown in table 6.2.

Some young women are anxious that if they drink the amount of milk needed they will put on weight. Women who are worried about gaining weight can choose from the many low-fat milks and dairy foods available that have all the nutrients and calcium as whole milk but without the fat. These will provide the calcium needed to build strong bones and reduce the risk of osteoporosis later in life.

Concern about today's diet

Concern about the kind of food we eat and its effect on our health has led to the establishment of expert committees in several Western nations. These committees have reviewed the information available and have produced reports in which 'nutritional guidelines' are recommended. Although the guidelines vary in detail and in emphasis, the recommendations are remarkably similar. Figure 6.1, the 'healthy diet pyramid', shows which foods we should eat most of and which we should eat least of.

For better health, teenagers and adults should modify their eating behaviour in the following ways:

- Choose a nutritious diet, eating a variety of foods from the five groups of food—breads and cereals; vegetables and-fruits; dairy products and protein foods such as meat, fish, and eggs.
- Eat more potatoes, pasta, and fresh vegetables and fruit.
- Reduce the amount of fat in the diet by avoiding fried and prepared foods. Remember: fat is hidden in cakes, biscuits, pastry, sausages, and rissoles. Eat more lean meat and fish and fewer fatty cuts of meat, mince, sausages, luncheon meats, meat pies, and pastries. This does not mean that you cannot eat hamburgers or other take-away foods. Most people, including teenagers, enjoy these foods. Just don't eat them too often!

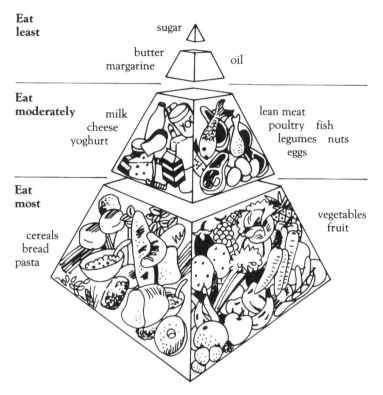

Figure 6.1 The healthy diet pyramid.

- Eat only moderate amounts of sugar.
- Avoid eating too many salty foods.
- Eat foods containing calcium.
- Eat foods containing iron.

This might sound a bit overbearing, but it isn't too difficult to keep to these guidelines (most of the time). It does not mean that you can't eat hamburgers, fried chicken, pizzas, ice cream, and chocolate bars or drink soft drinks. It simply means that you have to be sensible about your food choices, particularly if you are worried about gaining weight. You can avoid this if you are selective in the types of foods you choose and limit the quantity that you eat (see table 6.3).

Some young women who are trying to be very healthy and others who are worried about gaining weight adhere to these

Table 6.3 Good healthy eating

Eat more	Eat less
Whole grain breads and cereals	Confectionery (sweets, lollies, chocolates)
High fibre breakfast cereals	Cakes, biscuits
Legumes	Fatty meats and chicken skin
Potatoes	Butter
Vegetables	Salt
Fruit	Fried food and take-aways
Lean meat and poultry	High fat snack foods
Fish	
Low fat dairy foods or soy products	

guidelines. Unfortunately, they might be so concerned about their diet that they avoid nearly all fats and sugar and so might become undernourished and ill. It should be remembered that these are only *guidelines* and should not be taken to extremes.

Some teenagers become vegetarian in an effort to lose weight. Although eating a vegetarian diet will not cause malnutrition provided that milk, eggs, and cheese are included in the diet, it will not necessarily result in weight loss. Vegetarian diets are discussed later in this chapter.

Energy

Food provides both the energy needed to keep your body functioning and the nutrients to keep it healthy. Energy is expressed as kilojoules or kilocalories. A teenage woman requires between 8000 kJ and 9000 kJ per day (1900–2100 kcal per day) to meet her energy needs.

Selection of foods

For good nutrition a person needs to eat a variety of foods that provide adequate amounts of carbohydrate, protein, fat, dietary fibre, calcium, iron, and vitamins (such as folate and vitamin C).

Carbohydrate

In the past carbohydrate foods were classified as either simple or complex because of their chemical structure but this did not tell us about how these foods acted in the body. To understand more about the actions of carbohydrates we now describe their Glycaemic Index or the GI, that is how quickly or slowly foods are digested and absorbed into our blood stream. There are many factors that effect the time it takes to break down foods such as how it is cooked or how it is broken up or processed. The typical Western diet tends to be higher in refined carbohydrates with less whole grains and therefore has a higher Glycaemic Index; the food is broken down and absorbed more quickly. Examples of low GI food are dense grainy breads, basmati rice, pasta, noodles, rolled oats, and muesli. Sticky rice, processed breakfast cereals, smooth-textured breads, and some types of potatoes have high GIs.

The benefits of eating foods with a lower Glycaemic Index include a more sustained release of energy during the day, more stable blood sugar levels, and a reduced appetite. The GI of some foods is difficult to guess. Because sugar dissolves easily in water you might expect sugars to have a high GI, but not all sugars have a high GI; some sugars such as fuctose (fruit sugar) and lactose (milk sugar) are slowly digested and absorbed, so most fruits and dairy foods have a low GI.

Fats

We all need some fat in our diet, but most adults eat too much fat, particularly too much animal (saturated) fat. At present, fats provide 33 per cent of our daily energy requirements, and much of this comes from saturated fats. Nutritionists suggest that we should reduce the fats we eat so that they provide less than 30 per cent of our energy requirements, and that only 8 per cent of the energy we consume each day should come from saturated fat. This means that we should eat lean meat rather than fatty meat. We can eat poultry (but not the skin), and we should eat more fish, especially cold-water fish (such as salmon, trout, sardines, and mackerel). Fish contains essential fatty acids (omega

3 fats), which protect us from coronary heart disease, improve brain development in children, and help our immune system.

When possible we should not fry the meat, poultry, or fish but grill or barbecue it. Some fat in cooking will do no harm, particularly if unsaturated oil, olive oil or canola oil, is used. Unsaturated margarine (rather than butter) can be used on bread or buns.

Fibre

Fibre is thought to be important in preventing certain diseases. Most people in the developed countries eat too little fibre, and are more likely than people living in the developing countries to develop 'Western lifestyle' diseases. We eat only about 20 gm of fibre each day. We should aim to eat about 30–40 gm per day. The best sources of dietary fibre are shown in table 6.4. Recently, food manufacturers have become aware of the importance of dietary

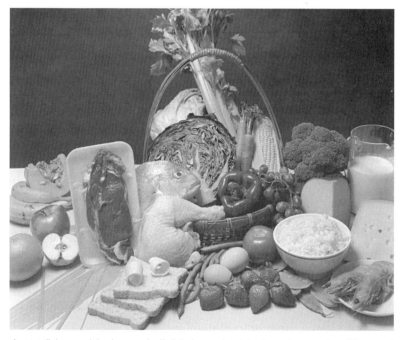

A sensible and balanced diet is important in keeping us healthy and helping us to feel good.

fibre and are now producing breakfast cereals that provide a quick and easy way to obtain fibre. As you can see from table 6.4, there are other ways of obtaining all the dietary fibre you need.

Table 6.4   Best sources of dietary fibre

Source	Average serving size	Dietary fibre
Breads and cereals		
All-bran	$\frac{1}{2}$ cup	9.5 gm
Muesli	$\frac{1}{2}$ cup	6.3 gm
Rolled oats, cooked	1 cup	3.4 gm
Whole-wheat breakfast biscuit	2 biscuits	3.2 gm
Unprocessed wheat bran	1 tablespoon	2.2 gm
Wholemeal pasta, cooked	1 cup	9.7 gm
Brown rice, boiled	1 cup	2.9 gm
Bread, wholemeal	1 slice	2.0 gm
Bread, white	1 slice	0.8 gm
Fruit		
Passionfruit	2	5.8 gm
Pear	1	4.3 gm
Apple, unpeeled	1 medium	3.1 gm
Banana	1 medium	3.1 gm
Vegetables		
Spinach, English	$\frac{1}{2}$ cup	4.6 gm
Sweetcorn	1 cob	4.0 gm
Peas, green	$\frac{1}{3}$ cup	3.6 gm
Carrot, peeled	$\frac{1}{2}$ cup	2.4 gm
Other		
Baked beans	$\frac{1}{2}$ cup	6.6 gm
Coconut, desiccated	$\frac{1}{2}$ cup	5.5 gm
Almonds	$\frac{1}{2}$ cup	3.8 gm
Sesame seeds	1 tablespoon	1.3 gm

Protein

Adults who are not ill need no more than 60 gm of protein each day, and teenage women need no more than 45 gm per day. As most teenagers enjoy eating foods containing protein, most will obtain all the protein they need for repairing tissues and keeping healthy. Table 6.5 lists the best sources of protein.

Table 6.5 Best sources of protein (you need 45 gm per day)

Source	Average serve size	Protein
Beefsteak, grilled	1 small rib steak	32 gm
Chicken, baked	1 half breast	25 gm
Fish	1 fillet	29 gm
Kidney beans	1 cup	12 gm
Cheese, Cheddar	2 slices	10 gm
Milk	1 cup	9 gm
Soy drink	1 cup	9 gm
Mixed nuts	½ cup	8 gm
Peanut butter	1 tablespoon	7 gm
Egg	1 medium	6.5 gm
Bread	1 slice	3 gm

Calcium

Teenagers need to eat and drink (as milk) at least 1000 mg of calcium a day because their bones are growing during the teenage years. Calcium strengthens bone and acts as a 'bone bank' to keep the bones strong as you grow older.

Iron

Red blood cells contain iron, and sufficient levels of iron in the blood are required to prevent anaemia (a lack of iron in the blood). Because women menstruate, during which time they lose blood, they must be careful to maintain their blood iron levels. Studies have shown that about 10 per cent of teenage girls are mildly anaemic. A woman needs about 15 mg of iron per day. The foods that are the best sources of iron are shown in table 6.6.

Table 6.6   Best sources of iron (you need 15 mg per day)

Source	Average serve size	Iron
Bran flakes (fortified cereal)	1 cup	8 mg
Liver	40 gm	4.4 mg
Beef	100 gm	4 mg
Lentils, chickpeas	1 cup	3.6 mg
Wholemeal pasta	1 cup	3.1 mg
Chocolate drinking powder	1 tablespoon	1.7 mg
Bread, wholemeal	1 slice	0.7 mg

Zinc

This important mineral is necessary for the formation of tissue in the body. It is part of the enzymes involved in the healing of wounds. Rich sources of zinc are oysters, red meats, veal and pork, nuts, and fortified cereals.

Folate

Folate is an essential vitamin and necessary to prevent anaemia and for the normal development of the brain and spinal cord of the baby before birth. Folate is contained in green leafy vegetables, peas, and lentils and to a lesser extent in spreads such as Vegemite and Marmite. Doctors consider this nutrient to be so important they recommend additional folate should be take by all women considering (or risking) pregnancy. Insufficient folate in the first three months of pregnancy is linked with defects in the development of the spinal chord, resulting in conditions such as spina bifida.

Vitamins

A large number of people take vitamin tablets to make them feel healthier. Most people obtain all the vitamins they need from the food that they eat and do not need supplementary vitamins, so the effect of the tablets is only psychological. A few teenagers may need extra vitamin C, and the rich source in fruit and vegetables makes it easy to obtain the 40–60 mg needed each day without spending money on vitamin tablets (see table 6.7).

Table 6.7 Best sources of vitamin C (you need at least 60 mg per day)

Source	Portion	Vitamin C
Orange juice	1 cup	125 mg
Grapefruit juice	1 cup	94 mg
Papaya (pawpaw)	$\frac{1}{2}$	94 mg
Melon (cantaloup)	$\frac{1}{4}$	56 mg
Strawberries	$\frac{1}{2}$ cup	42 mg
Potato (baked in skin)	medium size	30 mg
Tomato (raw)	medium size	28 mg

Some vitamins, especially vitamin B6 and vitamin D, are harmful if doses of 50 mg per day and 50 μg per day, respectively, are exceeded. Too much vitamin A (more than 7500 μg per day) causes liver and bone damage and other abnormalities. Pregnant women should avoid eating foods rich in vitamin A, such as liver and liver products, and taking vitamin A capsules. Excess vitamin A is particularly dangerous to pregnant women because it can cause birth defects in unborn babies.

Food myths

A good deal of nonsense is written about foods and eating. The problem is that people come to believe that they are right about their food beliefs and everyone else is wrong. This is because food, eating, and dieting receive such a wide exposure in magazines and books, on TV, and on radio talk-back programs. This makes it all confusing. The following is an attempt to highlight the facts—not the fads!

Myths about food

MYTH   Teenagers eat too much fast or junk food.

FACT   Many fast foods, for example hamburgers, are good foods (but not if eaten in excess). Some fast foods, for example confectionery (sweets, lollies, chocolate bars), contain hidden fat and sugar. They should be eaten sparingly.

MYTH   Sugar is bad for you; it is pure, white, and deadly.

FACT   Too much sugar is bad for you, but small amounts of sugar are OK.

MYTH   Although sugar is bad for you, honey is good because it is natural.

FACT   Honey is also sugar; it is no better for you than cane or sugar-beet. Small amounts of honey can be substituted for sugar, but not used in addition.

MYTH   Australian teenagers need to add salt to their food because of the hot climate.

FACT   Most people eat too much salt; extra salt is needed only if you do severe physical activity in temperatures above 40°C.

MYTH   Teenagers eat too much meat.

FACT   Too much for what? We eat more meat than we need to supply our bodies with protein, but that does no harm. What does harm is to eat too much fatty meat and to fry rather than grill meat.

MYTH   Starchy foods are bad for you.

FACT   Potatoes and bread (especially wholemeal bread) are good for you.

MYTH   Teenagers need vitamin tablets, especially vitamins B, C, and E.

FACT   If you eat adequate amounts of fresh fruit and vegetables you do not need vitamin tablets to be healthy.

MYTH   Vitamins relieve mental and physical stress, and prevent colds.

FACT   There is no evidence that vitamins relieve stress, except by making you believe they do. Vitamin C does not prevent colds.

MYTH   If a little amount of vitamin does you good, a lot will make you feel even better.

FACT   It won't. Excess vitamins B and C merely pass through your body and are lost in your urine or bowel motions. Excess vitamin A and D dissolve in your body fat and can cause illness. Excess vitamin B6 (pyridoxine) (more than 100 mg per day) can cause temporary nerve damage.

MYTH   'Processed' foods are bad for you as they have lost their goodness during processing.

FACT   Apart from losing fibre and perhaps a small amount of vitamins, processed foods have not lost their goodness. But they might contain too much salt and sugar. Read the labels on processed foods so that you know exactly what they contain.

MYTH   You should buy your food in a health food store rather than a supermarket because the food is healthier.

FACT   Most foods in supermarkets are as healthy and as good for you as most foods bought in health food stores. Some foods bought in both places are neither healthy nor cheap.

MYTH   If you engage in sport, especially swimming or running, you need extra protein and vitamin tablets to improve your performance.

FACT   There is no evidence that extra protein or vitamins improve performance.

A short guide to what teenagers should try to eat

Most teenagers know what they enjoy eating, but the following might help to choose a balanced, nutritious diet. Try to make up the food you eat from the five groups described in table 6.8.

Table 6.8   Five food groups

1   *Bread, pasta, rice, cereals, noodles*
    (Preferably wholemeal or wholegrain products)
    At least 4 servings per day
    1 serving   =   2 slices of bread
               = $1\frac{1}{3}$ cups of breakfast cereal flakes
               = $\frac{1}{2}$ cup of muesli
               =   1 cup of cooked rice or pasta

2   *Vegetables and legumes*
    4 serves per day
    1 serve   = $\frac{1}{2}$ cup cooked vegetables
             = $\frac{1}{2}$ cup legumes—dried beans, peas, lentils
             =   1 cup salad vegetables
             =   1 potato

3   *Fruit*
    3 serves per day
    1 serve   =   1 medium piece e.g. apple, banana, orange
             =   2 small pieces e.g. apricots, kiwi fruits
             =   1 cup canned fruit
             = $\frac{1}{2}$ cup juice
             =   dried fruit e.g. 4 dried apricots,
                 $\frac{1}{2}$ tablespoon sultanas

4   *Meat, poultry, eggs, fish, nuts, legumes*
    2 serves per day
    1 serve   =   2 eggs
             =   60-100 gm meat, fish, chicken
             = $\frac{1}{2}$ cup tinned fish
             = $\frac{1}{2}$ cup cooked (dried) beans, lentils,
                 chick peas, split peas

	=	$1/3$ cup peanuts or almonds
	=	$1/2$ cup sunflower seeds
5	*Dairy foods*	
	3 serves per day	
	1 serve =	1 cup milk
	=	40 gm, 2 slices cheese
	=	200 gm or 1 tub yoghurt
6	Other foods (providing energy but few nutrients)	
	1 to 3 serves per day	
	1 serve =	1 doughnut
	=	4 plain sweet biscuits
	=	1 slice plain cake
	=	$1/2$ small chocolate bar
	=	1 small packet of chips
	=	1 can soft drink

The diet in table 6.8 provides all the nutrients you need to keep your body healthy.

Teenage vegetarians

A number of teenagers decide that they will stop eating meat, fish, and poultry and become vegetarians. Provided alternative sources of protein, such as nuts and legumes are included as well as food from each of the other food groups, there is no reason why a vegetarian cannot be well nourished and healthy. It is not simply a matter of becoming vegetarian, however, because there are three types of vegetarian diet. All of them contain cereals, nuts, vegetables, fruits, legumes (peas, dried beans, lentils), and seeds. The three also include other foods.

The *lacto-ovo* vegetarian diet includes milk, cheese, yoghurt, and eggs. The *lacto vegetarian* diet contains milk and milk products but not eggs. The most strict vegetarian diet of all, the *vegan* diet, excludes all foods of animal origin, including eggs, milk, and milk products. The vegan diet is more risky to health than the other two as it is difficult to choose foods that balance each other nutritionally, and it is essential to take vitamin supplements (particularly vitamin B12). There are also some extreme vegetarian diets, for example the fruit-and-nuts diet or the Zen macrobiotic diet, which are potentially dangerous.

If you choose to be a vegetarian you can be as healthy as meat eaters and obtain all the nutrients you need, provided you choose your vegetarian diet sensibly. It is recommended that you consult a dietitian before you become a vegetarian.

Planning a vegetarian diet

First, make sure that you get enough protein of the right type. All proteins are made up of building blocks of smaller units called amino acids. There are twenty amino acids, eight of which cannot be made in your body and have to be supplied in food. These eight are called essential amino acids. Animal foods, including milk, yoghurt, cheese, and eggs, contain all the essential amino acids, but plant foods lack one or more of them. Fortunately, plant foods do not all lack the same essential amino acid, so if you mix the vegetarian foods you eat, you will make up your needs. You do not have to eat the same mix at every meal as long as you eat the different vegetable foods during the course of the day.

Second, you need to be sure that you get enough calcium. If you are a lacto vegetarian or a lacto-ovo vegetarian you will probably get enough, but if you are a vegan, you will need to eat nuts (especially almonds), soy beans, soybean milk, tofu, sesame seeds, and tahini paste. You also need to make sure you get enough iron and zinc in your diet. Non-vegetarians get their iron and zinc from red meat, liver, and kidney. As vegetarians do not eat these foods they have to choose their vegetables carefully to get enough iron and zinc. The best vegetarian sources of iron are wholegrain breads, fortified breakfast cereals, cashew nuts, legumes, whole grains, such as, bulgar and barley, and wholemeal pasta. The best vegetarian sources of zinc are legumes, eggs, cheese, and yoghurt. Vegetables and fruits are low on zinc, so a vegan has to eat a wide variety of vegetarian foods or she might become zinc deficient.

Third, vegans need to take extra vitamin B12 supplements (which have to be given by injection) or use a soybean milk containing added vitamin B12.

A suggested diet for lacto-ovo vegetarians

You have to choose from each of the four food groups (excluding the meat group), and the number of servings suggested is the minimum to meet your nutritional needs (see table 6.9). You might enjoy or need extra serves to meet your energy needs.

Table 6.9   A diet for lacto-ovo vegetarians

1	*Bread, pasta, rice, breakfast cereals*	
	(Preferably wholegrain cereals)	
	4 or more serves per day	
	1 serve	=	1 slice of bread
		=	½ cup of breakfast cereal, rice, pasta, or cooked porridge
		=	¼ cup of muesli
2	*Vegetables and legumes*	
	4 serves per day	
	1 serve	=	½ cup cooked vegetables
		=	½ cup legumes—dried beans, peas, lentils
		=	1 cup salad vegetables
		=	1 potato
3	*Fruit*	
	3 serves per day	
	1 serve	=	1 medium piece e.g. apple, banana, orange
		=	2 small pieces e.g. apricots, kiwi fruits
		=	1 cup canned fruit
		=	½ cup juice
		=	dried fruit e.g. 4 dried apricots, ½ tablespoon sultanas

Make sure you eat a serve rich in vitamin C every day (citrus fruit or juice, tomato, papaya (pawpaw), melon, cabbage, cauliflower, broccoli, brussels sprouts). The body easily absorbs the iron in animal products but not in plant foods. Vitamin C helps the body absorb iron from plants. Make sure you eat a serve rich in β-carotene (which converts to vitamin A in the body). This is high in carrots, pumpkin, spinach, silverbeet, broccoli, apricots, papaya, and melon.

4 *Eggs, nuts, legumes, seeds, 'textured vegetable protein'*
   2 serves per day

1 serve	=	2 eggs
	=	$\frac{1}{2}$ cup cooked (dried) beans, lentils, chick peas, split peas
	=	$\frac{1}{3}$ cup peanuts or almonds
	=	$\frac{1}{2}$ cup sunflower seeds
	=	2 tablespoons peanut butter or nut paste
	=	100 gm tofu
	=	100 gm textured vegetable protein

5 *Dairy foods*
   3 serves per day

1 serve	=	1 cup milk or soy milk
	=	40 gm or 2 slices cheese
	=	200 gm or 1 tub yoghurt

6 *Other foods (providing energy but few nutrients)*
   1 to 3 serves per day

1 serve	=	1 doughnut
	=	4 plain sweet biscuits
	=	1 slice plain cake
	=	$\frac{1}{2}$ small chocolate bar
	=	1 tablespoon of margarine
	=	1 can soft drink

Chapter Seven

Teenage eating behaviour and disorders

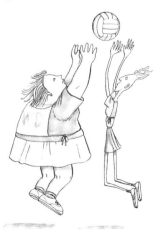

They are as sick that surfeit with too much, as
they that starve with nothing.

William Shakespeare, The Merchant of Venice

Historically, women were considered more attractive if they were plump. If you look at statues from Roman times, or paintings from the thirteenth century onwards, most women are portrayed as being plump. It was fashionable to be fat. There were several reasons for this fashion. First, food was often scarce and famines not uncommon. A plump person had body stores of fat to help her out during the lean periods. Second, if a woman was plump, it told the world that she was a good wife, as she must have a full pantry. Third, a woman's fertility was valued highly. From their experience of famines, people knew that badly undernourished women did not menstruate. Plumper women did menstruate, so plumpness was associated with the ability to produce babies.

Today, for almost the first time in Western history, women who live in the developing countries desire to be and to remain slim. To be slim is to be fashionable. This is not the situation in developing countries, particularly in southern Africa and the Pacific. This change in attitude is recorded in women's magazines, in fashion magazines, in advertising on television, and in the records of the 'vital statistics' of participants in beauty contests. If you look at the pictures of women who have won international beauty contests in the past twenty years and check their vital statistics, you will see that the more recent winners have been slimmer and taller than winners in earlier years. To be slim in countries where food is abundant and easily bought indicates that the person is disciplined, fit, healthy, and consequently desirable.

Another way of finding out whether women want to be thinner than they are is to check the numbers of new diets that appear regularly in magazines and in paperback books. The diets all claim to help you lose weight painlessly, effortlessly. If they were successful, new 'exciting' diets would not appear so regularly. And some diets are dangerous. They might damage your health.

Chapter 3 described the 'growth spurt' that precedes and overlaps early puberty. During the period of the growth spurt, teenagers eat more food because their bodies need more energy and this makes them hungry. After menarche the growth spurt ceases and her energy needs fall, but by now the teenager continues to eat the same amount as she has become accustomed to,

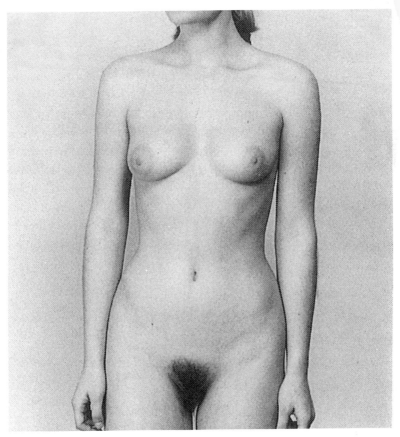

The shape of a typical teenager's body.

and this allows her to develop a more mature figure and lay down some reserves of energy. In the two or three years after her first period, the young woman may see this increase in weight as undesirable, and she may feel there is a big discrepency between the weight she is and the weight she wishes to be.

This is a teenage woman's dilemma. She might want to become slim or to remain slim to comply with today's fashion, but if she wants to control her weight, she has to control how much food and what sort of food she eats and how much exercise she takes.

Controlling weight by controlling eating and exercise seems simple in theory, but it is not so simple in practice. The genes inherited from your parents play a part in whether you will be fat or thin. Most women find that there is a body weight, their own 'set point' for weight, where they can remain relatively easily. When they overeat occasionally and vary the amount of exercise they get, their weight does not change much from their genetically programmed weight. However, there is a problem in contemporary society: the 'genetic' body weight and shape of most women is not as thin as is currently fashionable. If you want to have a body weight and shape that are below your genetic 'set point'-body weight, you have to remain constantly on a weight-reducing (restricting) diet. In other words, any increases in food intake (energy in) will result in weight gain towards your 'set point'. On the other hand if you are above your 'set point' and you eat less at any time your weight will drop towards your 'set point'

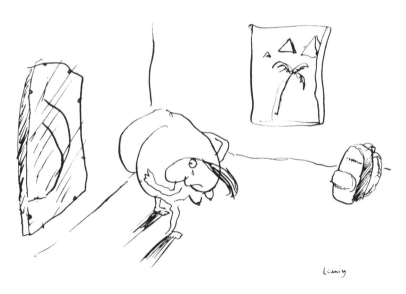

There is a further problem. People tend to write and talk about the energy (measured in kilojoules) and the nutrients we need each day because this is how nutritional scientists report their findings. This suggests that our bodies respond to and measure the amount of food we eat, and the energy it releases, each day. Why each day? A person's body responds (by changing in weight or shape) to the amount of energy consumed and expended over weeks, not days. If you become overconcerned about how much you eat each day, and become anxious if you vary that amount, even slightly, you might become depressed and start eating to cope with the feeling of depression. For example, you might say, 'I have eaten too much today so I have failed. I will eat some more so that I feel better.'

The biggest problem for most women wanting weight loss is not being able to reduce the amount and type of food eaten, but overcoming their bodies' messages to find food and eat in response to this deprivation of energy. This can lead to binge eating.

Most teenage women look at their bodies in a mirror and

Table 7.1 Areas of the body from which Australian teenage women want to lose weight

Area	% (1981)	% (1987)
Thighs	64	75
Bottom	45	65
Hips	43	80
Waist/stomach	22	80
Legs	20	
Face	9	
All over	9	
Breasts	6	
Arms	6	

want it to have a different shape. Many see their bodies as large and overweight compared with the idealised pictures of fashion models (see table 7.1). Many teenagers look at their bodies part by part. They observe the size and shape of their breasts—too big or too small or too floppy. They look at their bottoms. They look at their thighs and see them as larger and uglier than they are. The perception by a teenage woman of her body as larger than it really is occurs in many Western countries. (It can also occur in women who change their shape and size. For example, pregnant women often overestimate their size.) In an investigation in a town in Sweden, 26 per cent of 14-year-old women perceived themselves as fat, and more than half of the 18-year-olds thought they were fat. When the women's perceptions of their bodies were measured against the 'standard height and weight tables' for Swedish women, more than half the young women had over-estimated their size and shape. In the United States, a study of a thousand teenage women showed that they were particularly preoccupied with their body shape and their weight. Half the teenagers said that they were obese, but when their weight was measured against the 'standards' for American women, only a quarter of the women could be classified as obese.

In Australia, one in every ten women aged between 17 and 20 is overweight or obese, but one woman in five thinks that she is too fat. We asked Australian teenagers what they would like their body weight to be. Twenty women in every hundred were happy with their present weight, but the other 80 per cent wanted to be a little or a lot lighter. Some of the teenagers who wanted to lose weight were underweight when we talked with them; some were in the normal weight range and some were overweight.

Because of her perception that her body is fat and ugly, at least every second teenage woman goes on a diet or on several diets! She might keep to the diet, and if she does she will lose about 3 kg. She might stop and start dieting. 'Yo-yo' diets nearly always fail, and women using this method do not lose much weight; in fact, they usually end up gaining weight over several years.

Even if she keeps to her diet, she will have an irresistible urge to eat and might go on an eating binge. A large number of teenage women, whether they are dieting or not, go on eating binges. An eating binge occurs when a woman feels she cannot stop herself from eating a large amount of food, far more than she usually eats, over a short period of time, usually less than two hours. During the binge she might eat any kind of food, but often chooses foods rich in fat and sugar, such as sweets or lollies, ice cream, chocolates, cakes, and biscuits. She also chooses potato or corn chips (which are high in fat) and drinks sugary soft drinks. One teenage woman in every seven claims to have an eating binge once per week, and surveys in Australia, the UK, and the USA show that one teenage woman in three has an eating binge once per month.

Even if a teenager doesn't binge-eat she is likely to indulge in 'picking' behaviour. 'Picking' occurs when you go from the fridge to the cupboard or to the biscuit box eating a small amount of this and that, until you do not remember how much you have eaten. Picking behaviour and urges to eat lead to large swings in the amount of food a teenager eats each day. The size of the swing seems to increase in the week before the woman's menstrual period is due, although the amount she eats depends on how she feels that day.

From investigations in Australia, the UK, Sweden, and the United States, it appears that many teenagers diet, and more than half of teenage women have episodes of overeating when they feel they can't stop. In other words, they go on an eating binge. After an eating binge the teenager feels guilty; she looks at her body and worries about its size and shape. She might resolve to diet more strictly, to lose weight from her thighs, her bottom, her hips, and her waist, in that order. Fashion plays a large part in our lives. Fashion says that to be slim is to be healthy, to be beautiful, to be desirable, to be lovable. Most young women want these attributes, and they believe that to achieve them they must control the amount of food they eat.

Most teenage women are able to control how much food they eat, and, even with occasional binges and episodes of picking, manage to keep their weight in the 'desirable range', although it might fluctuate about 2 or 3 kg over a twelve-month period.

Some young women, especially if they want to be fashion models or dancers, aim to be thin and are a little underweight. Because of the need to keep thin they are rather preoccupied with their weight and their diets. Some common types of eating behaviour of such women are:

- avoiding eating between meals
- avoiding eating breakfast or other meals
- going on a diet, usually of their own design
- trying to eat only low-kilojoule foods
- avoiding being in places where there is food
- drinking water before a meal in order to feel full
- smoking cigarettes
- becoming vegetarian.

Other young women desire to be slim and try to diet, but often lose control. When control is lost the young woman goes on an eating binge, which usually only lasts a few hours but during which she might eat large quantities of food. After a binge she might feel awful and vow to keep rigidly to her strict diet or, less commonly, might learn to induce vomiting, either during or after the binge. A few young women abuse laxatives. These women have an eating disorder called bulimia nervosa, which is discussed later in this chapter. Two or three teenage women in every hundred have bulimia nervosa.

A few teenage women, probably about one in every 300, become obsessive about becoming fat. They have a fear that if they eat they will become fat. They start on a relentless pursuit of thinness. They refuse to eat or, if forced to eat, they vomit. Often they use other ways of avoiding food. They have anorexia nervosa (discussed later).

Some young women ignore the pressure to be thin or can't resist the urge to eat. They increase the amount of food they eat, they may feel better when they are eating and become fat. In studies in the countries we have mentioned, it appears that about 8 per cent of teenage women aged 14–17 are obese, and this percentage rises to 12 per cent in the 18–20 age group.

These then are eating disorders: bulimia nervosa, anorexia nervosa, and obesity. They are not illnesses in themselves. They become illnesses when they interfere with the teenage woman's life to a marked degree. They become illnesses when they upset the lives of her parents or close relatives. And, in severe cases, particularly of anorexia nervosa and bulimia nervosa, unless help is sought, the young woman might become very ill and might die. By the age of 19, one in two teenage women has dieted at some time, one in three has an occasional eating binge, one in seven has an eating binge once per week, one in eight is overweight, one in twenty-five is obese, one in forty has bulimia nervosa, and one in 300 has anorexia nervosa. Before discussing the eating disorders that might affect teenage women, it might help if we provide some helpful hints about overcoming these problems. These are listed in table 7.2.

Table 7.2 Eating problems and recommended solutions

Problem	Recommended solution
Women who eat only once or twice per day often become obese, because they gorge themselves when they do eat.	Eat something at least three, preferably four, times per day.
Daily fluctuations in body weight are not measures of body fat. Repetitive weighing usually leads to weight gain, as you respond to a tiny gain by eating more because you have 'blown' it and to a tiny loss (mostly fluid) by eating more.	Do not weigh yourself more than once per week.
Most people unknowingly overestimate (anorexia nervosa) or underestimate (bulimia nervosa) their energy intake.	Do not count kilojoules or calories.
Learn how much other people eat, at least at meal times, without causing a change in weight (remember: people eat at other times).	Eat with other people.
If you eat low kilojoule foods you become used to eating larger volumes of food. When you change to normal foods, weight gain can occur.	Do not preferentially select low kilojoule foods.
If you do not let yourself eat 'bad' foods you will frequently binge on them. This will occur even if you decide never to eat a food you consider 'bad'.	Try to stop thinking of foods as 'good' or 'bad'.
Your body weight depends on what you eat over weeks, not days.	Stop trying to control your food intake on a daily basis.
Body weight fluctuates for many reasons. A woman is considered to have a stable weight if she varies within 3.5 kg over a year. To try to keep your weight within 0.5 kg is unrealistic.	Do not try to stay at exactly the same body weight.

Problem	Recommended solution
The more you think about food and weight, the worse the problem becomes. Reading diets and recipes, counting kilojoules, and daily weighing are all likely to increase the preoccupation with eating and weight.	Stop doing things that keep you thinking about food and weight.
The greater the time spent preparing food, the more people eat. Preparing food keeps you thinking about food.	Spend the least time possible preparing food, cooking, and in the presence of food.
Trying to diet or starve is likely to lead to more binge-eating.	If you have a binge or bad session of 'picking', return to your normal eating pattern immediately.
Some women keep a private store of food at home (for security or as a test of self-control). You will eventually eat the food and feel bad.	Do not keep a private store of food at home.
There are no magic or instant ways of controlling or changing body weight.	Try not to fall for 'magical' or 'instant' cures.
Some theories of eating behaviour involve vitamin deficiencies, hormonal imbalance, hypoglycaemia, and allergies.	Do not fall for fashionable explanations of your eating behaviour.
Body shape is inherited, you cannot change it. Exercise, if substantial, can modify shape a little.	Take a realistic look at your body shape.
Are you trying to reach or maintain body weight that is too low for your body to stay at without constant dieting? Many women who choose careers requiring a low body weight have to battle to stay at these weights.	Take a realistic look at your body weight.

Problem	Recommended solution
Young women examine their body in parts. Older women look at the overall effect.	When looking in a mirror, look at the overall effect, not at parts of your body.
Many women regard exercise as a chore and either do not do any, or do not enjoy it if they do.	Choose a form of relaxation and exercise you enjoy and can maintain. Relaxation and exercise help most women feel better about themselves and their bodies.
Do you overexercise? Excessive compulsive exercising is a psychological disorder, and all you will be doing is exchanging one psychological disorder (eating) for another (exercise).	Do not exercise excessively.
Are you at a low body weight or not able to stop losing weight? Do you feel your eating is disordered and is affecting your life? Are you using dangerous methods of weight control? Do you use alcohol or drugs to prevent eating? Do you think you have a problem with food and eating?	Seek professional help.

The eating disorders

While most teenagers have no major problems with their eating behaviour—apart from an occasional binge—a few develop eating disorders. In the first type of eating disorder, anorexia nervosa, there is a considerable amount of weight loss, so that the person becomes extremely thin. In the second, which is called bulimia nervosa or compulsive eating, the person's weight is usually in the normal range, although the person might be overweight or underweight. In the third, the person is overweight or obese.

In many cases the eating disorders, particularly anorexia nervosa and bulimia nervosa, begin in the teenage years after menarche, when young women are experimenting and trying to control their body weight and shape. During the adolescent years, many teenage women experience periods when they are preoccupied with thoughts of food and body weight, and are concerned about controlling their weight and eating behaviour. Most teenagers pass through these periods with no problems, but for a few it is the beginning of an eating disorder. Often, the onset of the eating disorder is associated with a time of stress. Perhaps there are problems within the family, perhaps the teenager has a need to achieve independence, perhaps there has been the break-up of an important relationship, perhaps the pressure of study for an examination has been too great.

Although a person who develops an eating disorder usually develops only one of them, occasionally one can precede another or two might occur together. For example, some women who have anorexia nervosa have frequent episodes of severe binge-eating and are diagnosed as having both anorexia nervosa and bulimia nervosa. Other women who have had anorexia nervosa start putting on weight and begin binge eating, usually because they try to remain at body weights that are too low for them—some have bulimia nervosa and others become obese.

Anorexia nervosa

It is probable that a few women have starved themselves at all periods of history, but it was only in 1873 that an English doctor, Sir William Gull, used the term *anorexia nervosa* for voluntary starvation. He was looking after a young woman who was emaciated after losing 15 kg (33 lb) in weight. He could find no reason why she was so thin, and mistakenly assumed that her apparent lack of appetite (anorexia) was due to a 'morbid mental state' (nervosa). Sir William was a most experienced doctor, but he was wrong. Women who have anorexia nervosa do not have a lack of appetite. They are often hungry, but they suppress their hunger and refuse to eat normally because of their relentless desire to be thin, and because they are afraid that they will lose control of their eating behaviour and become fat.

In the years since Sir William wrote about anorexia nervosa, the number of people (particularly young women) affected by the disease has increased, and doctors have become more aware of its features. The first feature is that the woman is abnormally sensitive about being fat, or has a morbid fear of becoming fat, and of losing her control over the amount of food she eats. This fear induces her to adopt behaviour that she believes will help her to pursue thinness and to avoid gaining weight. Such behaviour includes dieting, excessive exercise, induced vomiting, and drug and laxative abuse.

Second, because of her fears and sensitivity about being fat, by the time she is diagnosed as having anorexia nervosa she has lost a considerable amount of weight and usually weighs less than 45 kg (99 lb or 7 stone). However, merely considering a level of weight that makes no allowance for the person's height or age is simplistic, and doctors now tend to use more sophisticated calculations. The simplest of these is a calculation called the body mass index (BMI). The index was used originally to define obesity, but it is equally useful for diagnosing anorexia in women over the age of 16 who have passed puberty. Before that age it becomes a bit inaccurate because of the growth spurt, and the BMI requires modification.

You can find your BMI easily. You have to weigh yourself in indoor clothing (without shoes) and measure your height. If you do this you can find your BMI by the following formula:

$$\text{BMI} = \frac{\text{weight in kilograms}}{\text{height in metres} \times \text{height in metres}}$$

A woman whose weight is in the normal range has a BMI between 19 and 24.9. If the person's BMI is between 18.9 and 17.1 she is underweight and, if other criteria we have mentioned are all present, she might have anorexia nervosa. If her BMI is 17 or below, the woman is emaciated and probably has anorexia nervosa. A BMI higher than 25 indicates that the person is overweight or obese (see table 7.3).

Table 7.3 The body mass index for women aged 15 or older

BMI	Description
40 or more	Severe or morbid obesity
30–39.9	Obesity
25–29.9	Overweight
19–24.9	Normal weight
17–18.9	Underweight
Less than 17	Emaciation

The third feature of anorexia nervosa is that a woman stops menstruating. Lack of menstruation is called amenorrhoea. As nine people out of every ten who have anorexia nervosa are women, amenorrhoea is a useful sign. Amenorrhoea can occur early in the illness, before the woman has lost any great amount of weight, and might persist for a number of months after she has been cured. When a woman's BMI is between 17 and 19, her periods usually stop and when her weight falls to a BMI of less than 15, they invariably do.

A doctor who uses these features to diagnose anorexia nervosa has to be careful. For example, a woman who has a severe mental illness might believe that someone is poisoning her food and refuse to eat, so that she loses a considerable amount of weight. Another example is that a woman who has terminal cancer, or a severe chronic illness, might become emaciated. While these illnesses can be differentiated from anorexia nervosa, in other cases it might be more difficult. For example, young women who are fashion models or ballet dancers have to remain at a 'fashionable' low weight (their BMI is usually between 17 and 18.9) because of their occupation. At times, when under stress or after an illness such as influenza, the woman's weight might drop to a BMI of 17 or less and she usually has amenorrhoea. If she sees a doctor she might be misdiagnosed as having anorexia nervosa. For these reasons, a woman must not have other physical or psychological illness that might account for her loss of weight, before a doctor makes the diagnosis of anorexia nervosa. The doctor must also take care that the weight loss, resulting from the illness, has not precipitated the woman into anorexia nervosa.

Pursuing thinness

Women with anorexia nervosa pursue their desire to be thin in several ways. Obviously most choose the simple way of drastically reducing the amount of food they eat; because of their preoccupation with body weight and food, they learn a great deal about food and food energy values. They cut down on, or stop eating, 'energy-dense' foods such as cakes, sugar, and sweets, and rich fatty foods. However, the diet they choose usually reduces all foods.

Because of their knowledge about food and energy, women who have anorexia nervosa frequently count the number of kilojoules (or calories) in their food. (Some even count the number of kilojoules in the piece of celery they are chewing!) They weigh themselves several times a day to make sure that they are not gaining weight. Many anorexic women avoid going to social outings where they know food will be served and where they will be expected to eat, in case their resolve not to eat is broken.

A woman with anorexia nervosa usually hides how little she eats from her family and her friends, and has several tricks to do so. She might move the food around on her plate to appear as if she is eating. She might put the food into a tissue instead of her mouth, or give it to the family dog under the table. She might take over the cooking for the family so she can control the amount of food she eats. She might prepare a big lunch to take to school or work, and throw it away when she leaves the house. Because her family believes she has eaten a large lunch, they accept that she wants to eat only a small amount at the evening meal. She might avoid family meals and eat with other people, so that they do not find out how little she really eats.

As well as avoiding eating, a woman who has anorexia nervosa might start exercising because she has learnt that if you exercise, you burn up energy more quickly. Some anorexic women devote many hours a day to exercise, and find it difficult to sit still. Exercise gives the woman an excuse to avoid food, as does study. Some women lock themselves in their room to 'study' and so avoid family meals.

Some anorexic women use dangerous methods of weight control, such as self-induced vomiting and the use of excessive amounts of laxatives. These do not work, but many anorexics do use them. These women usually do not reach extremely low body weights, are more likely to go out socially, and have a poorer knowledge of nutrition.

Anorexia nervosa patients are preoccupied with thoughts of food and body weight and with issues of control over their eating and body weight. Their obsession with their eating, weight and food allows little time for living a normal teenage life. Anorexia nervosa becomes an all-absorbing hobby to the exclusion of most other activities. Although the woman is aware that she looks thin, she feels fat. She will not perceive that she is as emaciated as she appears to others. She frequently denies her behaviour, and it might take time before she recognises that she has a problem. She might not be aware that she is experiencing swings of mood and is irritable with the family. It is only when she perceives that she has a problem, or the family perceives it, or she becomes dangerously ill that she seeks help.

Can anorexia nervosa be prevented? Anything that will help a young woman to stop losing weight, so that her weight is in her healthy weight range, will help her to avoid anorexia nervosa. A few young women describe passing through a brief 'phase' of anorexia nervosa when they were preoccupied with food, body weight, and dieting. This phase usually only lasts a few months after which the woman eats normally, as she has responded to the advice, comments, or threats of family and friends, and her weight loss has not been too excessive.

Some young women lose weight in an effort to feel healthy. They do this by not eating fat and by exercising. If too much weight is lost too fast, the teenager might be unable to gain weight and develop anorexia nervosa. These women need special help in hospital, sometimes for many weeks, if they are eventually to regain a normal lifestyle.

Bulimia nervosa

While anorexia nervosa patients love food but don't eat because of the fear of getting fat or losing control of their eating, bulimia nervosa patients have frequent episodes of compulsive eating when they eat large amounts of food. A woman with bulimia nervosa feels that she can't avoid what are called 'eating binges' as they are outside her control. Because of their love of food and of eating, women who have bulimia nervosa often call themselves 'foodaholics'.

Most people go on eating binges from time to time, so the fact that someone binge-eats is not enough to diagnose them as having bulimia nervosa. People who merely binge-eat return to their normal eating patterns after the binge, but women who have bulimia nervosa do not. A young woman who does not have bulimia nervosa might binge-eat at a time when she is dieting or is attempting to lose weight (and so is hungry) and on occasions because she likes food.

Women who have bulimia nervosa, on the other hand, go on frequent eating binges, often every day, sometimes many times per day, and at least twice per week. Usually, an eating binge lasts less than two hours, but the urge to binge might last for weeks. Bulimic women (and most bulimics are women) divide their days into 'good' days when there is no desire to binge-eat and 'bad' days when the compulsion to binge-eat is irresistible.

During an eating binge the amount of food the woman eats is excessive. In fact, *bulimia* means to 'eat like an ox', and some women who have bulimia nervosa do just that. On days of bad binge-eating, a bulimic woman might eat food that contains as much as fifteen times the energy needed by her body in one day. The type of food eaten varies from person to person and from binge to binge. Some binges might be high in carbohydrate, some in fat, and others in protein. Some women only binge-eat the food they describe as 'bad' and which they do not allow themselves to eat at other times; others will eat whatever is available, including what is in the rubbish bin.

Most bulimics say that an eating binge relieves their 'bad feelings', such as loneliness, anxiety, tension, and depression. Unfortunately the relief is brief, as the woman quickly feels 'bad' about her bingeing behaviour. This in turn leads her to binge again to relieve the bad feelings.

Many bulimics go to great lengths to try to resist the urge to binge-eat. The methods chosen vary considerably. Some women keep no food in the house, buying only what is needed each day; others avoid cooking or going into the kitchen. Still others avoid eating with the family or going out to social gatherings where food is served. A few women take more positive action by locking themselves in the bathroom, or driving into the country where no food is available, or keeping no money in their purse. Others try to divert their thoughts from food, planning to be completely occupied at all times, by knitting obsessively, telephoning friends, or going out to meet people. Some undertake work with long periods of overtime, in jobs where no food is available; others try to keep to starvation diets and avoid food shops. Other women use exercise as a way of avoiding binge-eating. They spend long hours at the gym, play squash or tennis, or jog for many kilometres each day. Some of these strategies are useful as long as they are applied sensibly. For example, drinking large amounts of coffee or caffeine diet drinks is not sensible.

When a bulimic woman goes on an eating binge she likes to do her excessive eating in private, and might become tense and angry if she is interrupted. Compulsive binge-eating can be such a secretive form of behaviour that the woman's family might not know for years that she has bulimia nervosa.

Women who have bulimia nervosa know that they will gain a considerable amount of weight if they go on binge-eating as often as they do. Because of this they attempt to avoid gaining weight, first by safe methods of weight loss, such as sensible dieting and exercise. When they fail to keep their weight down using these methods, they frequently resort to the more extreme and dangerous methods, such as starvation between binges or excessive use of laxatives, diuretics (fluid tablets), and slimming tablets, self-induced vomiting, and excessive exercise. Most bulimic women have tried many different methods of losing weight, and they are susceptible to any 'magical' method or the latest 'fad' that claims to result in quick weight loss.

Warning   If you are using any of these methods regularly, or a combination of them, it would be advisable to consult a doctor.

Women who have bulimia nervosa resemble women who have anorexia nervosa in many ways. They love food, and they are preoccupied with thoughts of food, eating, and body weight and with issues of control over their eating and weight. A bulimic woman experiences the same feelings of loss of control over eating that an anorexic woman fears might happen to her. This preoccupation interferes with the woman living a lifestyle appropriate to her age.

Unlike anorexia nervosa patients, only a few bulimic patients are thin; most are of average weight or are rather overweight. But most have wide swings of weight from thin to fat or fat to thin over relatively short periods of time. And like anorexia nervosa patients, many women with bulimia nervosa do not seek help for a number of years, or until one of the dangerous methods of weight control, such as self-induced vomiting, starvation, and laxative abuse, make her unwell or it becomes apparent to the woman's relatives that she is ill or she recognises that she is ill. When it is recognised that she is ill, medical help is sought.

The doctor will try to find out if the young woman has other signs of bulimia nervosa so that a diagnosis can be made and treatment offered. If the doctor discovers that she has had episodes of binge-eating at least twice a week for three months or more, and that she consumes large amounts of food during the binge, the diagnosis of bulimia nervosa can be made. It is important to stress that during the binge the woman must consume a large amount of food, because some women who have anorexia nervosa believe that eating a single chocolate bar is a binge.

It is also worth noting that women with bulimia nervosa do not use all of the dangerous methods of weight control. Some use one method, others use more than one method. We mention this because some teenage women and the media believe that unless she induces vomiting a woman cannot have bulimia nervosa. You can have bulimia nervosa and not cause yourself to vomit.

Binge-eating disorder

Women with binge-eating disorder resemble those who have bulimia nervosa. They have episodes of binge-eating, but these young women do not respond by severely restricting their food intake or purging in order to prevent or lose weight. As these women do not pursue thinness like young women with anorexia nervosa, they might increase their body weight and become obese. It is now thought that perhaps a third of adult women are obese as a result of binge-eating. The reason for this type of eating behaviour seems to be that the young woman has low self-esteem, feels that she is not as 'successful' as her peers in attracting other people, and might sublimate her discontent by eating large amounts of food at intervals.

Obesity

Obesity occurs when a person has, over a period of time, eaten food containing more energy than her body needs. The excess energy that she eats each day is converted into fat in her body, and slowly but surely she becomes fat. At first her weight is in the BMI range of 25 to 29.9. She is overweight. It is easier for her to lose weight at this stage. If she doesn't change her eating behaviour she will go on gaining weight and become obese, that is, her BMI will reach 30 or more. If she continues to eat more food than her body uses as energy, she will continue to put on weight and might become morbidly obese. Her BMI will now be 40 or more.

Obese people are more likely to develop gallstones, varicose veins, hernias, high blood pressure, and diabetes when they reach middle age, and breast cancer and arthritis when they become elderly. Morbidly obese people are at even greater risk of developing these diseases. Overweight people probably are not at risk, but all too often they become obese. There is a further reason for separating being overweight from obesity: obese people find it much more difficult to lose weight permanently than overweight people.

Many overweight and obese women try to lose weight; some are happy to be the way they are. A woman who has tried to lose weight might have dieted successfully at times but is unable to keep her weight down because she is unable to change her eating behaviour permanently. She likes and enjoys food. Many obese patients describe unpleasant reactions to being placed on low-energy diets. The main problems are a preoccupation with food, irritability, nervousness, and depression. These symptoms are similar to those voiced by women with bulimia nervosa and those who have anorexia nervosa.

Although the main reason why people become fat is because they consistently eat more energy than they use up, other factors can be involved. Many factors have been stated to be responsible for obesity, but research has shown that:

- There is no increased absorption of food from the gut of obese individuals compared with people of normal weight.
- Obese people do not lack the thyroid hormone, and in most cases there is nothing wrong with their glands.
- Obese people do not appear to have a greater 'addiction' than do thin people to sweet foods containing more carbohydrate.
- There is no compelling evidence that obese people choose a diet with a higher energy content than that chosen by thin people. Further, in an experiment, when obese individuals were given two foods of similar appearance, one of which contained a high energy content and the other a low energy content, they were unable to detect any difference in the two foods.
- There is no conclusive evidence that obese people are less active than thin people.

There is a possibility that a few overweight and obese people have an obesity gene (or genes). This is being investigated. An obesity gene might explain why some people who do not appear to eat much food become obese: they are 'programmed' to use the energy they absorb from food more efficiently than thin people can. This means that people who will become, or who are, obese use less energy for any given activity, including their body functions, than thin people, and the excess of energy obtained from food is converted into fat and stored. It is important to note that for all but the most active people, sedentary activities (which includes the body's resting metabolism) account for most of the daily energy expenditure. It is possible that obese people are genetically programmed to be more efficient in handling this proportion of their energy expenditure, although they use the same proportion of energy for exercise as lean people (see table 7.4).

Table 7.4   Energy expenditure for certain daily activities

Activity	kJ per kg per hour	kcal per kg per hour
Sleeping, lying still awake	4.0	1.0
Sitting quietly, eating, watching TV, reading, studying	6.3	1.5
Dressing, undressing, washing, preparing food	9.6	2.3
Walking slowly, driving a car, clerical or secretarial work	11.7	2.8
House cleaning, walking at a moderate rate	13.8	3.3
Playing table tennis, cycling, walking fast	20.1	4.8
Ice-skating, dancing, playing tennis or netball, horse-riding (trotting or galloping), skiing	25.0	6.0
Vigorous exercise during a competition	32.0	7.8

However, the explanation for the recurrence of obesity in certain families could be due to the family's eating behaviour rather than to their genes. Fat parents might have fat children (and fat pets) because the family members enjoy food and are big eaters: food and eating are perceived as socially pleasurable and desirable.

Another theory is based on the observation that an obese person has a larger number of fat cells in her body than a thin person. When faced with the challenge of fat to be stored, the fat cells first increase in size and then, when a critical size is reached, divide to form new fat cells. Once formed, the fat cells never disappear. If a person continually eats more energy than she uses up, in every period that weight is gained an irreversible increase in the number of fat cells occurs. These fat cells in turn are able to store more energy in the form of fat, and the person becomes increasingly obese. Once a person has become obese, particularly if severely obese, it is difficult for her to lose weight because of the large number of 'hungry' fat cells that 'demand' to be filled. In some way messages reach her brain stimulating her to eat more.

The reasons why fat people become and remain fat are poorly understood, but most people accept that if you eat more energy than you expend, over the years you are likely to become fat. For example, if you ate 1260 kJ more energy each day than you expended, and if the net gain of this energy was 420 kJ (after allowing for the increased energy loss due to increased heat production), a net gain of 153,000 kJ would occur each year, which is equal to 2 kg (4.2 lb) of fat. Recently, increasing evidence has shown that human behavioural factors in eating control are important in the regulation of body weight.

You might be overweight and happy, but many teenagers are not. If you are unhappy you should seek professional help. It is available. If you are unhappy, losing weight will not cure the cause of your unhappiness, but it might contribute to feeling better about yourself. It is also useful to know that it is easier to lose weight if you are overweight than if you are obese. Only minor changes in what you eat might be sufficient. These minor changes might be as simple as using less margarine or butter, eating a piece of fruit instead of a piece of cake, buying fewer chocolate bars or lollies, stopping putting sugar in tea or coffee, avoiding thick milk shakes, and cutting all the fat off meat. Increasing the amount of exercise you do will also help. It also helps to take action in the teenage years, as four out of every five obese teenage women will be obese in middle age.

Help for eating disorders

Anorexia nervosa and bulimia nervosa

If you have anorexia nervosa or bulimia nervosa and are prepared to accept help, it is available. If you don't use dangerous methods of controlling your weight (self-induced vomiting and the use of laxatives and diuretics), you could get help from a community group or from your doctor. If you do use the dangerous methods, you need to see a doctor, at least initially. There is no set pattern of treatment, as different women respond to different approaches to treatment. Different approaches are also needed if the woman has problems in addition to an eating disorder. The currently popular term for this treatment is 'cognitive behavioural therapy' (CBT), although a lot more than CBT is involved

The general aims of treatment are to help the woman learn:

- what is normal eating behaviour
- to keep her weight in the healthy range, without having to resort to dangerous methods of weight loss
- to reduce her preoccupation with body weight and shape
- to establish a normal healthy lifestyle for her age.

To be successful the woman must be motivated to change her behaviour, and the advantages of getting better must be greater than the advantages of having the eating disorder. For many women the eating disorder must become extremely severe and have disastrous effects on their lifestyle before they are ready to get better. Some of the perceived advantages of having an eating disorder are described in the last section of this chapter. Recovery might take many years, during which lapses could occur. Most women find it helpful to have a professional person whom they can contact when lapses occur.

Obesity

If you are overweight, and particularly if you are obese, you might want to seek help. Many teenagers who think that they are (or are in fact) overweight rush off and buy a book, or read a magazine article that tells them how they can lose weight quickly, easily, and painlessly. As diet books appear with such great frequency, replacing an earlier 'guaranteed success' diet, you can be sure that most of them don't work for most people most of the time.

Teenagers often try to lose weight by avoiding eating the kind of food they like. But if you choose a weight-reducing or slimming diet, it has to be easy to follow. It has to permit you to eat many of the things your friends eat but in smaller amounts. It has to be a diet that you can continue eating for as long as you wish, without getting bored. And you have to remember that the only person who can make you keep to your diet is you.

You need motivation to keep to a diet, because there is no instant magical method of losing weight. It is easy to lose between 3 and 6 kg relatively quickly, but it is hard to prevent the return of that weight unless you keep to your weight-reduction diet. Permanent weight reduction is a slow process, and you should expect to lose no more than 0.5kg per week. Even if you do lose this amount of weight, you might find that your weight fluctuates from day to day, so don't weigh yourself more than once per week.

You should avoid going on a 'crash' diet. Although you might lose weight rapidly for two or three weeks on a crash diet, most of what you lose during that time is water stored in your muscles, and most is lost in the first week. After two or three weeks you will be so bored with the diet that you will abandon it and gain weight rapidly, as you regain the fluid you have lost.

A menu plan (see chapter 6) alone is not enough to help you lose weight and, once you have lost weight, to keep you at the lower weight. To lose weight successfully and permanently, a woman has to want to change her eating behaviour, and this requires more than a diet. Several things help you to keep to a sensible eating plan, and you can choose what you think will help you from the following list:

- Don't gorge by eating one large meal a day. You will lose weight more quickly and feel better if you eat several small meals spread over the day.
- Try to eat your meals at about the same time each day.
- When you have a meal, eat slowly.
- Before you start eating, decide how much of what food you will put on your plate, and don't add more. Once you start eating it is too easy to say to yourself: 'I'll just have a little more.' 'Littles' add up to a lot.
- It might help to use a smaller plate, so that the plate looks fuller.
- Once you have finished what you decided to eat, leave the table (if you can do so without offending anyone). If you stay at the table where there is food you might break your resolve not to eat any more.

- Don't keep a private stock of sweets or chocolate bars. You will be tempted to eat them.
- Don't raid the fridge.
- Take enjoyable exercise regularly, particularly after meals (see table 7.4). Regular exercise burns up energy and helps you to lose weight.

If you keep to these conditions and choose a menu plan that is easy to follow, you will lose weight.

Maintaining your lower weight

It is difficult to lose weight so that it lies in the range you desire; it is even harder to maintain your weight at the new level. Many people try to do so and find that, as their weight goes up and down, they try to overcome this by yo-yo dieting. Unfortunately yo-yo dieting does not work very well, and the woman's weight tends to go up. When you have reached your target weight, you will need to continue with the same new behaviours and attitudes to food and eating. At this time it is probably easier to see a dietitian who can look at your menu plan and work with you to help you maintain your achievement.

Perceived benefits of having an eating disorder

As eating disorders cause so many problems and need so much motivation, time, and effort to be cured, it is surprising that some young women believe that there are some benefits in having an eating disorder. We asked a number of young women with anorexia nervosa what benefits they thought having anorexia nervosa gave them. Below is a sample of their answers:

- 'You look fragile so people treat you gently and don't expect so much of you.'
- 'Because you look sick others look after you.'
- 'You have achieved what others cannot.'
- 'Controlling my food intake makes me feel in control of my life.'

We asked the same question of women who had been diagnosed as having bulimia nervosa. This is what three of them said:

- 'Binge-eating relieves bad feelings.'
- 'Food gives me "the rush" to make me high and happy.'
- 'Eating helps me cope with other problems.'

Finally, we asked obese women if they thought that there was any benefit in being fat. Two responded:

- 'I feel part of the family. They are all overweight.'
- 'People talk to me about their problems because they can see I am not perfect.'

Chapter
Eight

Adolescent sexual behaviour

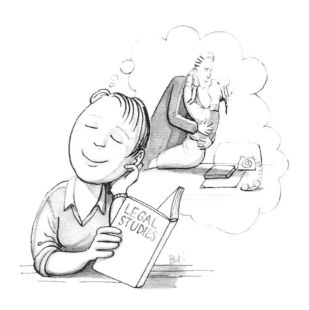

Love is like the measles; we all have to go through it.

Jerome Klapka Jerome

Some people still believe that it is only since the 'flower power' generation of the 1960s that teenagers have become sexually active outside marriage. This is not true. Some teenagers have been sexually active in all generations. For example, in the nineteenth century many young people engaged in sex, particularly in the rural areas of England and in the slums of the cities. In parts of England, young men were encouraged to 'taste before they bought'. In other words, it was usual for a young couple to have sex and, if a pregnancy resulted, to marry. In the cities, in the nineteenth century, child prostitution was far more common than it is today.

In the moralistic climate of Victorian England (and of Victorian Australia) this type of behaviour was not mentioned, and the 'respectable' middle class believed it only occurred among the poor. However, there is now evidence that a veneer of respectability disguised the licentious behaviour of many middle-class men who professed to be pillars of society.

Middle-class parents in class-conscious Victorian England were particularly sensitive to any suggestion that their daughters were sexual beings. Young women were not expected to have sexual thoughts, as they might lead to masturbation, which, it was believed, would damage their health and make them sterile. Young middle-class women were expected to be virgins when they married (although it was accepted that their husbands might have had previous sexual experience). If an unmarried middle-class woman became pregnant, she was regarded as a 'fallen woman' whose disgrace shamed her family and who had little hope of marrying unless the father of the child married her.

A young woman's sexual purity was of great concern. The predatory nature of men and the weakness of women was stressed in novels and in magazines. For example, *The Girl's Own Annual*, which had a large circulation, ran a column called 'Answers to Correspondents'. This was the predecessor of the 'agony aunts' of today's magazines and newspapers. In 1887, the *Annual* contained the following answers, which gave moral advice to young women.

Young Girl—At your early age (fifteen years) the less you read in the way of novels the better. Better be satisfied with history and travels, in the brief space of time free for recreation in the way of reading. In any case, we can only say in such matters, consult your mother. If she sanctions your reading any particular work of fiction, well and good. She will probably allow you to read those in prose and verse by Sir Walter Scott.

A Fearful Night—The two girls must have known it to be a disgraceful proceeding to receive two young men into the house, and encourage them to remain there till late, unknown to their parents; otherwise, they would not have concealed it from them. No blessing could rest on such clandestine meetings. Nay, their characters are already tarnished in the opinion of anyone who may have heard of it; and they must also hold a very low place for dignity and maidenly propriety in the estimation of the young men themselves.

Five-feet-nine—With reference to sending a young man a Christmas card, wishing 'the compliments of the season' in return for one from him, we can only say, consult your mother. She knows who he is, and all the circumstances of the case; we are strangers to all.

Agatha—You should not pray for a husband. How do you know that it would be for your happiness or your advantage, and not a hindrance to your usefulness and your spiritual life? Perhaps the field of labour which God designs for you is your parents' home. Pray rather that He would clearly point out the work for which He knows you most suited, and to give you wisdom, strength, and grace to do it. May He deign to employ you in however humble a vocation for His glory, as His faithful servant. If He deem you competent to fulfil the duties of a married woman worthily, and have no work for you to do at home, he will provide a suitable husband for you in His own good time. Acting on your own responsibility you cannot expect His blessing.

Pup—Taking walks with men, more especially in the evening, is not proper, unless you have a married or middle-aged woman always with you on such occasions, and your mother approves of the acquaintance.

Sans Souci—Can hardly expect us to advise her respecting the 'quickest and cheapest way to become an actress'. Even if good actresses were made in a 'quick and cheap' manner 'without paying a premium', as our correspondent says, we could not advise any girl to take up a career so full of temptations, struggles, and anxieties. There is no doubt that we are often called by God to positions where we have great temptations; but if so He will find us grace, and make a way to escape, that we may be able to glorify Him in our lives. Be content to choose some less dangerous career. We have no right to place ourselves in questionable positions and in difficulties, to which we are not called by a Divine Providence.

Letters from young women, seeking advice from 'agony aunts' 100 years later had certainly altered in content and tone, as had the advice. These two letters and their responses were published in *Cleo* in 1991:

ATTRACTED TO GAY GUY

Q I met a man at a barbecue recently who I'm incredibly attracted to. We've become friends, but I want more. He has now told me he is gay. Can a gay man ever be attracted to a woman and become straight? Reader, Vic.

A *I suspect he has revealed to you he is gay because he is well aware that you are attracted to him and he doesn't want to mislead you. In these circumstances, you should respect his honesty and not be so arrogant as to assume you will be able to 'convert' him to heterosexuality. This can only happen if the man is capable of experiencing attraction towards women as well as men. As you get to know your friend better, I am sure he will reveal to you whether he is capable of showing this type*

*of versatility in his sexual/emotional make-up. You will then
know if there is any possibility of a more intimate relationship
developing between you. But don't push it, or you will lose that
valued friendship in the process.*

SPRINGING CHRISTMAS SURPRISE ON PARENTS

Q My boyfriend wants me to go on holidays with him at
Christmas. I'd really like to, but it would be the first time I
haven't spent Christmas at home. Also, my parents don't know
we are sleeping together, and if I tell them that we're going
away, they'll guess. I don't want to upset them at Christmas.
Should I lie and say we are going with friends? Reader, Qld.

A *Don't kid yourself that your parents don't suspect you are
sleeping together. Most parents choose not to know their children are involved in a sexual relationship. If you flaunt the
issue in their faces by blatantly going away together, you force
them to acknowledge it and either endorse your sexual relationship or come out actively against it. Remember, it's likely
that your parents indulged in similar behaviour when they
were young. Now, as parents, they will feel a natural desire to
protect you from all the difficulties they know can arise from
early sexual activity—unwanted pregnancy and possible health
risks plus all sorts of emotional upheaval. It is natural that
many parents choose to stick their heads in the sand and just
hope for the best. I believe it is sensible to accept their feelings
and go along with this game. Find some friends to go with you
so your parents feel more comfortable. And, if possible, try to
be home for Christmas day. The festive season is not a good
time for your parents to have to deal with this unsettling issue,
let alone to deprive them of your company.*

Sexual activity among young people increased throughout
the first twenty years of the twentieth century, but the most
marked increase occurred in the 1920s, when middle-class
women were partially liberated from the constraints that had

kept them under full male control, first by their father and after marriage by their husband. More young women were sexually active when your great-grandmothers were adolescents than when their mothers were adolescents, and this trend has continued: when they were young women, more women of your grandmothers' era were sexually active than when their mothers were young, and still more women of your mother's generation were sexually active than when their mothers were young. Continuing this trend, a larger proportion of today's teenagers are sexually active, and it is true that their first sexual experience is occurring at an earlier age.

Sexual attraction

Sexual desire is a powerful urge. Once the sex hormones begin to be secreted into a girl's blood after puberty, she begins to have sexual thoughts and feelings. Her sexuality might be that she is attracted to another person. It might be that the other person arouses her sexually. It might be that she responds sexually. Obviously, unless she is attracted sexually to another person, she usually isn't going to engage in further sexual activity.

Why one person is attracted to another is not understood. But it happens, in real life as well as in romantic novels. In the latter, the attraction is often expressed in such terms as: 'Suddenly across a crowded room, Emma saw him—tall, handsome, rich, and she knew ... !' That quotation does not explain why Emma was attracted to Sir Reginald Maltravers, in the best romantic novel tradition. One theory that seeks to explain sexual attraction is that from early childhood each person develops her or his own sexual arousal pattern. This pattern is rather like the script or scenario for a TV series, but it is 'written' by the person and the person is the 'heroine' of the series. The scenario is based on childhood experiences, memories, and fantasies.

As the girl grows up, she adds to the script, rejects part of it, modifies part of it, rewriting it again and again in her subconscious mind until, after puberty, she has developed a script that describes the person or people to whom she is attracted sexually. She might modify the script as she grows older, and tinker with it throughout her life, but the people to whom she is attracted tend to be similar in many ways.

When she meets the type of person she has created in her scenario, she becomes sexually excited, and if the excitement is reciprocated by the other person (who has also developed his or her own scenario), the couple make closer contact. During this contact, which can extend over hours, days, or months, the couple explore each other's personality and, if they find they like each other, become closer, seeking to learn more about each other, or they separate because the initial excitement fails to be sustained. In the arousal scenario, four of the senses—sight, sound, smell, and touch—are involved to a greater or lesser extent. The other person's appearance is not just very important; at the beginning of the relationship it might be all-important. In other words, his appearance is more important than his intelligence or his status in society. But although appearance is important, sexual excitement is increased by the other senses. In many animal species, particularly birds, males go on display to attract females. This is not so obvious in humans, but most women would agree that the way a man dresses can be a strong attractant. The sound of a man's voice might attract a woman or repel her; so might his smell, whether natural or due to other scents, such as soap and cologne. For many people the touch of body contact is the most sexually exciting of all the senses. Most people feel sexually warm if they touch, kiss, or hug a person who arouses them sexually.

If the experience of all these senses confirms that each person really is sexually exciting to the other, and their personalities seem to be compatible, the couple might wish for closer intimacy. But how close that intimacy will be depends on each person's sexual values, attitudes, and beliefs; in other words, on their sexual behaviour.

Boyfriends

Adjusting to and coping with sexuality occupies a good deal of an adolescent's time. While most teenagers adjust well, some find it difficult. Having special male friends is important to most teenage women. But some teenagers worry and wonder why they do not have a boyfriend. The reasons are complex, and it is probably better to ask yourself 'How can I get a boyfriend?' rather than 'Why do I not have a boyfriend?' or ask 'Why do I want a boyfriend?'

How do you 'get' a boyfriend?

- You have to be ready to want to have a boyfriend. This might sound silly but it isn't. If you are not ready, you will give messages to people and it will turn them off. For example, if you feel you should have a boyfriend only because most of your friends have one, but you are shy, uncomfortable, or anxious about going out with a man, those messages will be conveyed in your body language. Body language, in which the other person learns about your feelings more from how you behave—what eye contact you make and how your body responds to what the person is saying—than from what you say, is important in developing a relationship.
- Don't set your goals too high. If your ideal man is a rock star or a soap opera hero, rich, handsome, and famous, you are very unlikely to meet him—except in the distance at a concert or in your fantasy life, when it can be fun!
- You don't have to look like a TV star, a model, or a sex symbol to get a boyfriend. Most people who have any real feelings for their partner want someone they are comfortable with, not an object for others to admire.
- You won't get a boyfriend unless you feel confident enough to go to places where you can meet males. The man in your fantasies who drives up and knocks on your door exists only in your dreams.
- It helps if you can learn 'social skills': being able to talk with people, feeling relaxed when you are with people.

- Join groups that have similar interests to your own, such as sporting, music, or art groups.
- Learn to like yourself. Think of what you are good at. Perhaps you are a good listener or a considerate person. If you feel you have no good points, you are wrong. Everybody has good points. Write out a list of your ten best points. For example, you might write 'I am a good listener'. Don't add '… but I find it hard to talk to people'.
- Letting a man have sex with you freely won't get you a boyfriend. Generally, all you will achieve is a series of one-night stands or very short relationships. If that is all you want, OK, but remember that the chance of getting a sexually transmitted disease is fairly high, and one-night stands usually don't lead to lasting relationships.

How do you end a relationship?

Usually, it is better for you if you end a relationship when you feel it's over than if your boyfriend ends the relationship. There is no one way to say 'goodbye'. Some relationships end, and the couple are able to remain friends; others end in anger and/or bitterness. When ending a relationship, however, remember that the other person has needs and feelings of his own; respect those needs, be sympathetic, and try to discuss your reasons for ending the relationship. Try to stand your ground and not give in to his pleadings for 'one more chance' as this is usually stressful and prolongs the suffering for both of you.

What to do when your boyfriend says it's over
- Contact your friends.
- Keep busy.
- Do things that make you feel good.
- Go out—even if it's by yourself.
- Remember: the pain and emptiness fade with time.
- Don't blame yourself.

Sexual behaviour

'Sexual behaviour' means ways of showing one person's love for another, of relieving sexual tensions, and of enjoying a shared experience. Types of behaviour range from sexual dreams to sexual intercourse. Some are solitary in nature, some need a partner. With sexual behaviour go sexual rights or freedoms and sexual obligations.

Sexual rights or freedoms

To be in control of your body and to reject sexual exploitation
That means to be able to say 'no' as well as 'yes'. If a man says: 'Unless you let me make love, you don't love me', a woman has two answers if she doesn't want to make love. The first is 'OK'; the second is: 'If you do make love, I'll know you don't love me'. If the man then says: 'If you really loved me, you'd let me', the woman could then reply, 'If you really loved me, you wouldn't want sex when you know I don't'.

To make your own sexual choices
This means to weigh up the 'fors' and 'againsts' and make a decision that you feel is the most suitable for you—provided that your decision does not exploit another person.

To refuse to be sexually stereotyped
That means to refuse to be told that women do this or do that sexually without being able to deny these claims.

To know about sexual myths
Myths by definition cannot be truths. In all human behaviour that is treated as 'secretive' or 'shameful', myths begin. Belief in some sexual myths can damage your sexual health, so if sexual matters are being discussed, try to decide whether it is a sexual truth or a sexual myth that is being talked about. Some common myths are mentioned later in this chapter.

Sexual obligations

Sexual freedoms and sexual rights need to be balanced by sexual obligations. Liberty is not license. Some sexual obligations are particularly important because of the damage they can do if they are ignored.

A person has the following sexual obligations:

- the obligation *not* to exploit another person's body sexually or commercially
- the obligation *not* to conceive an unwanted child, or cause another person to conceive an unwanted child
- the obligation to permit another person her or his sexual preferences
- the obligation *not* to impose her or his sexual preferences on others
- the obligation *not* to spread, or pass on, a sexually transmitted disease.

How do adolescents behave sexually?

It is difficult to find out how adolescents behave sexually because many people feel that to be asked questions about their sexual behaviour is an invasion of their privacy. Sex is usually a very private matter. When a person boasts about his sexual successes (and it is usually a man), the chances are that he is exaggerating in the hope of making his friends believe he is more sexually active and successful than he really is. In most Western nations, there has been a trend towards greater sexual freedom among teenagers. But there has been no reduction in the desire of most people for love and commitment in a relationship, and most people expect to marry some time.

The best organised studies of sexual behaviour have been made in the UK, Sweden, and the United States. There are considerable differences between the countries, between the two sexes, between individuals within each sex, and between young women and young men in different social classes.

Myths about masturbation

- Women do not masturbate.
- Masturbation is a sign that a woman cannot form a good relationship.
- Excessive masturbation causes weakness and physical illness.
- Women who need a vibrator are oversexed.
- Married women do not masturbate.
- In pregnancy, masturbation can cause an abortion or bring on labour.
- Masturbation might make a woman sterile.

Kissing, touching, and fondling

A couple increase their sexual excitement by touching, exploring, and stroking areas of the body, particularly those areas that are perceived as erotic. Although any part of the body can be erotically arousing, most women enjoy kissing, having their breasts fondled, having their genital area fondled, or fondling their partner's genital area. Most men are aroused by having their genitals fondled or when they fondle a woman's breasts and genital area. Touching can be limited to fondling through the clothes or the exposed breasts may be fondled or kissed, and the exposed genitals may be stimulated by the other person's fingers or lips. The stimulation might cause the person to reach orgasm. How many teenagers enjoy this sexual behaviour? Studies show that 85 per cent of young women aged between 15 and 19 have engaged in kissing and fondling and the average age for commencing these activities is under 15. Not all female teenagers enjoyed it; some did it only to please the males.

These sexual activities relieve sexual tension and if each partner is sensitive to the other's feelings, it also helps them both to develop their sexual knowledge. It gives them the opportunity to explore each other's bodies, including each other's genitals. It helps them to communicate with each other sexually, each telling the other what makes them feel good and what they don't like. It makes them more sensitive to each other's sexual needs and more receptive to their own sexual response.

Oral sex

Some couples obtain great sexual pleasure from oral sex. This is when a man licks a woman's clitoral area and when a woman sucks a man's penis. Some people condemn oral sex as unnatural. Although this belief must be respected by the other partner, surveys show that many couples regularly enjoy oral sex. Some people believe that oral sex is dirty, but oral sex transfers no more, or no fewer, germs between the couple than does kissing.

Some women who engage in oral sex are worried about what will happen if they swallow the man's semen when he ejaculates in the woman's mouth. The answer is that it is safe to swallow semen, although it has a distinctive taste. But if a woman does not like sucking the man's penis she should tell him. This is one of the sexual rights mentioned earlier in this chapter. Once told, the man has an obligation to accept her choice.

Sexual intercourse

Teenagers need to decide when to have sexual intercourse, with whom, and in what circumstances. Sexual intercourse is the penetration of the vagina by a man's erect penis. When a male is sexually aroused, his blood pressure increases slightly and blood flows to his genital region, causing the engorgement of the soft tissues of the penis, which increases in size and becomes erect. This is called an erection. In females, sexual arousal causes the engorgement of the clitoris and/or erectile tissues just outside the hymen but within the entrance to the genitals and deep within the skin. In addition, two pea-sized glands, known as Bartholin's glands, which are deep in the backward part of the vestibule, secrete mucus and moisten the entrance to the vagina so that the penis can enter it without discomfort. The thrusting motion made with the penis stimulates orgasm in the male—when his sperm is ejaculated (he 'comes')—and in the female, because of the motion of his penis against her clitoris and vagina.

Of all the sexual behaviour engaged in by adolescents, sexual intercourse arouses the most anxiety among parents.

Masturbation is accepted by many adults as normal behaviour for today's teenagers, kissing and fondling is permitted, but sexual intercourse between unmarried adolescents continues to be a matter of considerable concern to parents and to teenagers. Some parents accept that their children will have sexual intercourse, but point out the possible problems. These are that the girl might become pregnant and that if either partner has had one or more previous partners, he or she might give the current partner a sexually transmitted disease, unless he uses a condom or both partners agree to be tested to find whether they have a sexually transmitted disease.

Many parents, however, disapprove of adolescent sexual intercourse, particularly if they have a daughter. This creates a dilemma for many adolescents. If the parents of the teenager have attitudes to sexual intercourse that differ considerably

---

Myths about sexual intercourse

- The only proper way to have intercourse is with the man on top.
- If the woman is on top, it shows that the man is weak and the woman is a nymphomaniac.
- A woman cannot become pregnant if she has intercourse standing up.
- Pregnant women lose all interest in sex.
- In the first quarter of pregnancy, sexual intercourse will cause an abortion.
- In the last weeks of pregnancy, sexual intercourse will bring on labour prematurely and might harm the baby.
- If the man has sexual intercourse lying on top of his pregnant partner he will damage the baby.
- If a woman does not have an orgasm she will not get pregnant.
- As women grow older they lose their desire for sex.
- A woman who does not have an orgasm simultaneously with the man is frigid.
- A man can tell by the shape of her hips whether a woman will be good in bed.

from those of her peers, the young woman has to make a choice. Only the teenager herself can decide what is right for her; but to make this decision she needs accurate information about sexuality and relationships. Will she adhere to her parents' values or to those of her friends? If she chooses to do what her friends do, she might feel guilty about deceiving her parents; if she chooses to accept her parents' values, she might be rejected or mocked by her friends.

There are a number of myths about sexual intercourse that, if believed, can make your relationship less pleasurable. These myths are listed on p. 143.

Anal sex

In this the man inserts his penis in the woman's anus and rectum. It was believed that only homosexual male couples obtained sexual pleasure in this way, but information has become available that as many as 20 per cent of heterosexual men enjoy anal sex. For a woman anal sex can be painful and not enjoyable, and no woman should be forced by a man to have anal sex.

Beliefs about sexual activity

In 1966, an American sociologist found that most people held one of four beliefs about sexual activity, particularly sexual intercourse. They believed in one of the following: sexual abstinence, the double standard, permissiveness with affection, and permissiveness without affection. These four beliefs are discussed below.

Sexual abstinence

Those people who believe in abstinence think sex before marriage is wrong for both sexes, although some degree of kissing and touching might be permitted. Studies have shown that about 25 per cent of teenage women believe in sexual abstinence for themselves, but not necessarily for other teenagers.

The double standard

People who believe in the 'double standard' of sexual behaviour believe that men have a stronger sexual drive than women and need to satisfy the drive (or it might cause physical damage!). For this reason men can have sexual intercourse when they want. A woman, on the other hand, should be a virgin when she marries or may have sexual intercourse with her fiancé if she is engaged. The problems about the double standard are: (1) that there is no evidence that men have a stronger sexual drive than women; and (2) acceptance of the double standard implies that intercourse is a mere physical activity in which there is no obligation on the man to make sure his partner enjoys the sexual encounter. The double standard also allows adults to differentiate between 'bad' boys and 'bad' girls. A 'bad' boy is one who may fight excessively, steal, play truant, or take drugs. He is not 'bad' if he has sexual intercourse. To say a girl is 'bad' usually means that she is sexually active.

The double standard of sexual behaviour is still strong today. It causes problems for teenage women, who have to walk a narrow path. If they refuse to have sex, they are considered 'frigid'; if they have sex they are mocked as being 'slags' or 'sluts'. During the 1970s, studies showed that about 27 per cent of teenage men and 23 per cent of teenage women believed in the double standard of sexual behaviour. No studies have been made recently, but it seems that the proportions may have not changed significantly, although some men are receiving messages about acceptable sexual behaviour towards women.

Permissiveness with affection

People who believe in this sexual behaviour say that if the couple have an affectionate, relatively stable relationship, sexual intercourse is permitted. In other words, sex is OK if you have a good relationship. The relationship might last a long time or a short time, but during it neither partner has another sexual partner. If, or when, the relationship breaks up, one or both partners might form a new relationship. In this type of sexual behaviour, the woman expects the man to be considerate of her needs and to accept the sexual obligations and freedoms discussed earlier in this chapter. These relationships are referred to as serially monogamous relationships; and become more common as teenagers grow older.

Permissiveness without affection

People who believe in permissiveness without affection say that sexual intercourse is a pleasurable activity for men and for women, and each should be able to enjoy sexual intercourse because of the pleasure, regardless of the amount of affection between the couple. People who believe in this form of sexual behaviour tend to be 'sexual adventurers', that is, they are not interested in a sexual relationship but enjoy having several sexual partners, either simultaneously or serially. Today it is likely that about 20 per cent of women choose this type of sexual behaviour.

To describe a person as a sexual adventurer does not necessarily mean that she or he behaves in this way all the time. Some people are sexual adventurers for short periods of time. A person might become a sexual adventurer because she feels lonely or depressed. She might have sex with a number of men as she tries to be comforted and feel close to someone. She might be a sexual adventurer because she is angry with her family and wants to get her own back. She may have been abused as a child. Or she might become a sexual adventurer because she enjoys sex.

Changes in patterns of sexual intercourse among teenagers

Surveys in Australia and several other Western countries show that more teenagers are having sexual intercourse, and at an earlier age. Teenage men are more likely to have had sexual intercourse than teenage women, and teenagers of working-class parents are more likely to have sex at an earlier age than teenagers of the wealthier groups of society. The studies also show that the longer a person continues to be educated, the later he or she is likely to have had the first experience of sexual intercourse. In round figures obtained from surveys in the UK, USA and in Australia, 26–35 per cent of teenage men and 20–35 per cent of teenage women had had sexual intercourse before they reached the age of 16. By the age of 17, the proportions had increased to between 40 and 50 per cent of men and 40–45 per cent of women. By the age of 19, 80 per cent of teenage men and 75 per cent of teenage women had had sexual intercourse at least once.

The British survey also asked the teenagers the reasons for having sex. A quarter of the teenage men said it was 'natural', and a third said it was because they were curious. The reasons

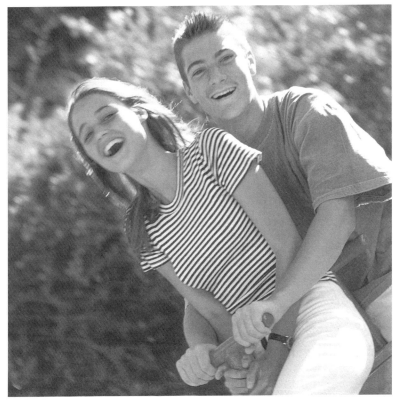

Most people want a loving, caring relationship with a special person.

that the teenage women had sex were rather different. Forty per cent said it was because they were in love, and 30 per cent said it seemed natural. The surveys show that most teenagers see nothing morally wrong in premarital sexual intercourse, and an increasing proportion of teenage men and women are sexually active at an earlier age. Chastity is no longer considered a virtue by many teenagers.

Early experiences of sexual intercourse

For sexual intercourse to be fully satisfying (except occasionally, when a brief sexual encounter might be very pleasurable), most women (and some men) prefer to be aroused by caressing, kissing, stroking, and touching before sexual intercourse is attempted. These activities are called 'foreplay' or, preferably, 'pleasuring'. They are not only pleasurable but also increase the moisture of the woman's vagina, making penetration by the man's penis more comfortable. Many women obtain sexual pleasure if the man strokes or licks the woman's clitoral area either before or after sexual intercourse, especially when this is the way she most often reaches orgasm. Most women and many men wish to continue in close intimacy after orgasm, enjoying a warm sexual after-glow.

This is the idealised version of sexual intercourse. The reality, especially in the first experiences of sexual intercourse, can be rather different. Most sexually active teenage women are worried about having sexual intercourse, at least for the first few times.

Several surveys have tried to find out how teenagers felt about their early sexual encounters. The most common problem reported by teenage women after their first experience of sexual intercourse was guilt, and more than half of the teenagers surveyed said they had felt guilty about having sex, although the guilt usually diminished after a few sexual encounters. Most of those who felt guilty had been pressured into having sexual intercourse, or had wanted to wait for sex until they were older and in a long-term relationship or married. Regret and guilt are more commonly reported among young teenagers. The younger the woman when she first had sexual intercourse the more likely it was to have been unwanted or involuntary (see chapter 11, 'Sexual abuse').

The next most common problem was disappointment—sex wasn't all that good. Linked with this was anxiety that the young woman 'wasn't good at sex' or 'didn't respond like women are said to do when you read women's magazines'. In other words, she was worried about her sexual performance because she didn't know what was 'normal' or if there was 'a right way' to have sex. Some teenage women were worried that if they 'weren't good at sex' and didn't give the man enough pleasure, he would break off the relationship and find someone more experienced. Other teenage women were worried because they didn't reach orgasm during intercourse. The myth that both partners should have a simultaneous orgasm is still strong. A few women were so tense and anxious that they found the first intercourse painful, and most didn't really enjoy the experience. The bad feelings and the anxiety were less if the man was loving, caring, and took time to make love.

For most teenagers the bad feelings decreased as their sexual experience increased; with additional experience, their anxiety about sexual performance, the guilt, and the discomfort were either reduced or ceased altogether.

Teenage attitudes to sexual activity

Most teenagers today begin sexual activity at an earlier age than the teenagers of past generations; they appear to enjoy a wider variety of sexual activity, and most teenagers do not feel guilty about having a sexual relationship. Surveys made in Australia and the UK show that most teenagers do not think it is morally wrong for people to enjoy sexual intercourse before they are married.

But most teenagers expect to marry and they want to marry, usually when they are in their middle twenties. Most do not believe that motherhood is the only career for a woman. Most agree that a woman should have the choice of having a job outside the home as well as caring for the house and children. And most want a marriage in which both partners share the homemaking and childcare responsibilities.

Dishonesty in dating

When a man tells you that he loves you and you alone, and only wants sex if you want it, is he telling the truth? Unfortunately he might well be lying. A 1990 investigation in the USA of 422 sexually active college students showed that a third of men aged between 18 and 25 had told a lie in order to have sex, and about the same number had lied about their ability to control their ejaculation. A third had lied about not being sexually involved with more than one female, and nearly half said that they would understate the number of previous sexual partners they had had.

If this dishonesty in dating occurs in other countries—and it probably does—you need to beware. It is possible that your potential partner has acquired a sexually transmitted disease, and either he doesn't know he has it or, if he does know about it, he isn't going to tell you about it. The two most common diseases are *Chlamydia* and herpes (see chapter 12). He might have acquired *Chlamydia* and did not know about it, but he can be tested for the presence of the organism. He should tell you if he has had an attack of herpes recently. (If the herpes is quiescent you are probably not going to be infected.) If he doesn't tell you about this sort of thing, you won't have much of a relationship.

Most sexual partners do not have a sexually transmitted disease, but if you have any doubt and you choose to have sex, it is worth protecting yourself by insisting that your partner uses a condom.

The 1990 study mentioned above did not investigate whether women lie about their sexual behaviour to men, but they probably do!

Teenage pregnancy—the facts

The USA

- In the USA more than a million teenage girls become pregnant each year.
- Four out of ten girls will become pregnant at least once before they are 20 years old.
- Half of teenage pregnancies occur within six months of first intercourse, because the couple did not use contraception.
- Since the late 1980s seven girls in every hundred aged 15–17 became pregnant each year.
- More than half of these girls had the pregnancy terminated by an abortion.
- The younger the teenage girl, the more likely she is to be anaemic, to miscarry, or to give birth to a low-weight baby.

Australia

- In Australia four girls in every hundred aged 15–19 become pregnant each year. As in the USA, the pregnancy is terminated by an abortion in 40–50 per cent of cases.
- A quarter of the girls will become pregnant again while still a teenager.

Adults' views of teenage sexual behaviour

Many adults believe that most teenagers have had sexual intercourse before they reach the age of 20. They are right. Adults also believe that most teenagers are sexual adventurers. They are wrong. The studies show that more than 50 per cent of sexually active teenage men and more than 60 per cent of sexually active teenage women have had sex with just one partner.

Most of the teenagers who had had or who were having sexual intercourse had been going out with (dating) the person for more than six months. Most adults believe that once a teenager has had sex she goes on having sex all the time. This is not true. Many adults also believe that the pill has led to the increase in teenage sexual behaviour. This belief has been investigated in several surveys, and there is no evidence that the pill has encouraged either casual or non-casual sexual relationships.

Adults also seem to believe that most sexual encounters between teenagers take place after a party, in a car, or at a hotel. The evidence is otherwise. Most teenagers have sexual intercourse 'at his place or mine', and his place is used twice as often as her place.

Some adults believe that if a 'young, immature' person has sexual intercourse it will lead to an 'irresistible impulse' to which the teenager rapidly becomes addicted. From this it follows that teenage sex is inevitably bad. The evidence from the surveys contradicts these beliefs. In one of the British surveys, 40 per cent of those who had sexual intercourse repeated the experience within a week, 50 per cent within two weeks, and 60 per cent within four weeks. However, 20 per cent did not have sex again for at least three months.

However, some teenagers enjoy frequent sex for pleasure or because they need money to pay for drugs. Forty per cent said it was because they were in love, and 30 per cent said it seemed natural.

The hazards of early sexual intercourse

The information presented shows that a large proportion of adolescent men and women have had sexual intercourse before they reach the age of 20. Once the couple have overcome their early experiences, sexual intercourse is pleasurable and produces a feeling of enjoyment. It is seen as an appropriate way of expressing intimacy.

Sexual intercourse, however, has hazards. The first is that the woman can become pregnant. As we discuss in chapter 9, unwanted pregnancies can be avoided if the woman uses a reliable method of contraception. The most reliable contraceptive for teenage women is the pill.

The second hazard is that unless action is taken, sexual intercourse can lead to sexually transmitted diseases. Unless you and your partner have had no other partners, the man should use a condom. Condoms prevent unwanted pregnancies but are not as effective as the pill. However, they are much more reliable than the pill in preventing the spread of sexually transmitted diseases. In the Netherlands many sexually active teenagers use the 'double Dutch' method of contraception, whereby the young woman takes the pill and her male partner uses condoms. This is the ideal, providing protection from pregnancy and sexually transmitted diseases.

Homosexuality

Homosexuality means that the person has an emotional and sexual preference for a person of her or his own sex. Female homosexuals (also called 'lesbians' or 'gay women') prefer to be intimate socially and sexually with other women, although they might have many male friends.

The number of lesbians in Australia is unknown, but probably about one woman in every fifty is gay. A lesbian might have had a relationship or several relationships with men, but decides that she is more comfortable with, relates better to, and is 'turned on' by, another woman. Apart from preferring other women sexually, lesbians do the same jobs, have the same interests, and take part in the same recreations as heterosexual women. Most lesbians are indistinguishable from heterosexual women, but a few act out by being aggressive and loud, and behaving as many men behave.

Because gay women pleasure each other sexually mainly by cuddling, kissing, and enjoying oral sex, they are less likely to acquire a sexually transmitted disease than heterosexual women or homosexual men.

Many teenage women develop 'crushes' on other teenage women or older women. This does not mean that they are gay, as most will become interested in men as they grow older. Women do not choose to be lesbian. A woman is not born a lesbian, nor is a woman necessarily always going to be a lesbian.

Being gay is not due to 'bad' genes or to a hormone imbalance. Nobody knows why some women are, or become, gay.

Some people believe that a lesbian is psychologically abnormal. This is a myth. Gay women have no more emotional problems than heterosexual women. There is no evidence that by enjoying the company of a gay woman, you will become gay yourself. Most gay women are gentle and considerate about the feelings of other women. Some women who have been married and have children later become gay. Children brought up by a gay couple are no different emotionally or sexually from children brought up by heterosexual couples. In fact, because the relationship between the gay couple is loving and because they touch each other often, the children's emotional development is likely to be better than that of a child whose parents fight or are distant to each other.

Gay women have all the feelings, emotions, needs, and desires of heterosexual women. They are not 'deviant'. But it can still be difficult for a gay woman, having made her decision, to 'come out' and tell her parents. It might also take time for her parents to accept that their daughter is gay. Given patience, most parents eventually accept that their daughter is a lesbian, and with this acceptance their relationships are loving and supportive.

Lesbianism—the facts

- It is not abnormal to be lesbian. Two per cent of teenage women are lesbians.
- Most lesbians have a full and enjoyable life.
- Alas! Some sections of society still believe that it is evil to be lesbian, and discriminate against lesbians.

Chapter Nine
Preventing pregnancy

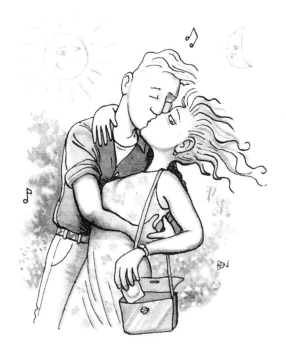

I must say ... a fast word about oral contraception. I asked a girl to go to bed with me and she said 'no'.

Woody Allen

When a man ejaculates, he releases more than 300 million sperm from his penis, and their intent is to succeed in making the 12 cm journey, propelled by their tails, through the uterus to reach the place in the Fallopian tube where the egg is to be found. But of the 300 million, only a few million will reach the uterine cavity. Of these, only a few thousand will survive the journey through its cavity, and only a few tens will enter the Fallopian tube down which the egg is passing. Only a few survive the journey up the tube, and only one penetrates the wall of the egg.

Nevertheless, in spite of the odds against a sperm reaching and fertilising the egg, statistics show that for a young woman who 'takes a chance' on having intercourse without using contraception, there is a high possibility that she will become pregnant. Sexual activity should involve respect for each other, it should not be exploitive; and it carries with it the responsibility of taking the necessary precautions against pregnancy and the spread of sexually transmitted diseases. In other words, a young woman should know about and consider using a contraceptive.

Even today it is not always easy for a young woman to obtain accurate information about contraception. Information is given out in schools (formally and informally), in families, and in magazines, but the most powerful medium—television—has avoided providing information until recently. If you watch television you see that sexual advertising is used to sell alcohol, cars, popular soft drinks, soap, menstrual protection, ice cream, and chocolate bars. Television offers instant intimacy, simulated violence, and music permeated with sex and sexuality. Advertising on television has for years extolled the use of pain-killers, laxatives, cough mixtures, worming tablets, and treatments for piles (haemorroids), but it is only since the AIDS epidemic that condoms have been advertised. Television could provide respectability for other types of contraception and information about preventing pregnancy.

Teenagers and contraceptives

At present one in four sexually active teenagers does not use contraceptives in the first few months of being sexually active, and after this time some still do not. There are a number of reasons why sexually active teenage women are reluctant to use contraceptives, particularly in the first months of sexual activity. The first is the belief by some young women that a sexual encounter should be spontaneous and 'romantic'. The teenager should be 'carried away by the passion of the moment', and taking precautions to protect herself against a pregnancy would make the experience planned and unromantic. Allied with this is a belief that a pregnancy 'cannot happen to me'. It can.

A second reason is that some teenage women do not want their parents to know they are having sex. If they have purchased packets of the pill or condoms, the packets might be found by one of their parents.

A third reason for not obtaining contraceptives is that as the pill can only be obtained on prescription, the teenage woman has to visit a doctor to obtain it. Some young women are reluctant to admit to a doctor that they are sexually active and want the pill, as they don't know what his or her response will be and whether or not the doctor will be judgmental and give a lecture about avoiding sex. There is, however, an alternative way of obtaining the pill. Rather than going to the family doctor, a teenage woman could choose to go to a family planning clinic or ask a family planning clinic (or friend) to recommend an appropriate doctor. Family planning clinics are staffed mostly by women, the atmosphere is pleasant, and all the advice is given in a non-judgmental manner.

Of course, the woman could buy a packet of condoms from a pharmacy or supermarket, but this might be embarrassing, as the assistant would know that the woman was sexually active. Condoms are available from vending machines in some women's toilets and change rooms and in most men's toilets and change rooms.

Facts of intercourse and pregnancy

- Women become pregnant because they have sexual intercourse.
- It is not romantic to be 'carried away' and have sex without using contraceptives—it's stupid.
- An excellent contraceptive is to say 'NO'.
- If he says he won't love you unless you let him have sex with you, he doesn't love you.

In the past, teenage women explained that their ignorance about contraception was the reason why they did not obtain contraceptives. (This reason is heard less often today.) Many parents were reluctant to talk to their daughters about sex and contraception, schools did not have classes in human sexuality, and magazines did not publish articles about contraception. The reason appeared to be that many parents and educators believed that if teenagers knew about contraceptives, more would become sexually active. This belief is false for two reasons. First, teenagers learn about sex and contraceptives from their friends anyway; second, teenagers have sex because they want to, not because they know more about it. More information about contraception does not increase promiscuity, but it does reduce the number of unwanted pregnancies. The advent of the AIDS epidemic has permitted a much more open attitude to sexuality and to contraception.

Another reason why some teenage women do not protect themselves against a pregnancy is that they subconsciously (or consciously) want to become pregnant. There are several reasons for this. The young woman might want to escape a family who do not seem to care about her or her needs, who constantly criticise her behaviour, who have problems that occupy most of their time and exclude her, or who are brutal to her. Teenage women brought up in such families often have a poor opinion of themselves and low self-esteem. By giving herself to a man and having his baby, such a young woman might believe that he will love her and she will have a happy relationship or, even if he refuses to stay with her, he will have given her a baby on whom she can lavish the love she misses.

None of these reasons is good. It is better to prevent a pregnancy than to become pregnant and have an abortion or give birth to a child who is not really wanted. Knowledge about contraception *does not* increase teenage sexual experimentation or activity, and contraceptives *do* prevent unexpected, unwanted pregnancies.

Contraceptives are not 100 per cent effective. A few teenage women become pregnant because the contraceptive has failed. The pill is the most effective contraceptive and rarely fails, provided that it is taken exactly as the manufacturer recommends; that is, the pill should be taken at the same time every day, starting on the first day of menstruation. If the woman vomits, or has a stomach upset or an episode of diarrhoea lasting for more than two days, the pill might not be absorbed properly, and a few medications (some antibiotics and vitamin C powder) also alter the absorption of the pill. In such cases, other contraceptive measures should also be used until seven active (see Page 168) pills are taken over the following seven days.

Condoms have a rather higher failure rate. The man might not have put the condom on properly, he might mistakenly believe you do not need to put them on until halfway through intercourse, or he might not have held it correctly when withdrawing after ejaculation and so let some sperm escape into the woman's vagina. Occasionally the condom 'bursts' during sex, but this is very uncommon. There is no truth to the myth that one condom in a hundred is pricked, but some teenagers still believe this claim.

Pregnancy prevention, contraception, and family planning involve having the information to be able to make choices. In an 'ideal' society, every sexually active couple could make sure that both partners understand all the options available and that one or the other is using a contraceptive before they start having sex. Unfortunately it is not an ideal world, and many men expect the woman to be taking or using a contraceptive. In spite of this, it is important for teenage (and adult) men to be aware that they have a responsibility to ensure that an unwanted, unwelcome pregnancy does not occur.

For this reason we will first discuss contraceptives used by men. Teenage men have two choices of contraception. The first is 'withdrawal', and the second is to wear a condom.

Contraceptives for men

Withdrawal

Withdrawal is a very old method of family planning, and in some communities it is a popular method. It depends on the man being very aware of when he is about to ejaculate ('come') and withdrawing his penis from the woman's vagina beforehand, making sure that when the semen spurts out of his penis it is well away from the woman's vagina.

The problem is that the man has to have learnt when he is about to ejaculate, and has to be sufficiently agile to withdraw quickly. A further problem is that, sometimes, a small quantity of sperm-rich semen might seep out of the penis before the man feels that he is going to ejaculate. These problems mean that the method is not very efficient (unless the man is practised), and pregnancies do occur.

Condoms

Modern condoms are made of thin latex rubber, coated with silicone, and sealed individually in aluminium foil packs. The man waits until he has an erection, then he unrolls the condom along the length of his penis. He makes sure that no bubble of air is left in the closed end, by squeezing the tip of the condom, or all of it, before he unrolls it. If the couple prefer, the woman can put the condom on the man's penis. The condom must be fully unrolled to the base of the man's penis. Otherwise, when the man's penis shrinks after he has ejaculated, the condom might come off, releasing sperm into the woman's vagina. Because of this risk some doctors recommend that the woman put some spermicidal cream (to kill any sperm that might escape when the man withdraws after ejaculating) into her vagina when her partner uses a condom. Most teenagers do not accept this advice for obvious reasons. It is difficult for the woman to have a tube of spermicidal cream with her, it disrupts love-making, and it makes sex seem premeditated. Many teenagers like sex to seem romantic or spontaneous.

Condoms have several advantages for teenagers. They can be bought from pharmacists without prescription and, in many places, from vending machines. They have no side effects, because no hormones or chemicals are used. This is because a condom prevents a pregnancy by creating a 'barrier' that prevents the sperm reaching the cervix.

If a man has had several partners (or if his partner has had several partners), which increases the risk of catching a sexually transmitted disease, the condom protects each partner from being infected by the other.

If a couple use condoms properly every time they have sex, only three women in every hundred will become pregnant in any one year.

In rare cases and after using condoms for a long time an allergic reaction can occur in the tissue of the vagina and be uncomfortable for a time. This is an allergic reaction to the latex of the condom.

How to use a condom
Refer to figure 9.1.
- The condom should be put on the erect penis before the penis is put in the vagina.
- Squeeze the tip of the condom for a length of 1 cm.
- Roll the condom all the way to the bottom of the penis.
- After intercourse hold the condom as the penis is withdrawn.
- Withdraw the penis soon after intercourse because if the erection is lost inside the vagina, the condom might slip off, spilling sperm.
- A condom can be used only once.

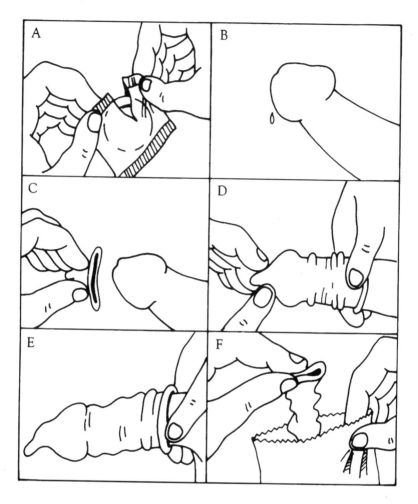

Figure 9.1 How to use a condom. (a) Open the packet carefully, and do not unroll the condom before putting it on. (b) Semen can leak out soon after the penis becomes erect, before ejaculation. To prevent pregnancy or infection, the condom must be put on before any sexual contact takes place. (c) Ensure that the condom is the right way up. Squeeze the teat on the tip of the condom, and hold it against the tip of the penis. (d) Unroll the condom all the way to the base of the penis. (e) After ejaculation, the penis should be withdrawn before the erection is totally lost. When withdrawing, hold on to the condom. (f) Do not allow the condom or penis to come into contact with the female's genital area, and carefully dispose of the condom.

How to keep the condom

Good-quality condoms keep for about two years if stored away from heat. Don't keep condoms in your pocket for more than a few days as your body heat could damage the rubber.

Advantages of using condoms

- A condom effectively protects the woman from an unwanted pregnancy, provided that the condom is used properly each time the couple has sexual intercourse.
- The condom effectively protects each sexual partner from acquiring a sexually transmitted disease, and it is more effective in doing so than any other form of contraception (except abstinence).
- The condom can be bought from a variety of sources and does not need a doctor's prescription.
- Women and men can buy condoms.

Possible disadvantages of condoms

Studies in several countries show that not all men who are sexually active, and particularly if they are 'sexual adventurers', use condoms regularly, although the numbers are increasing. There are two main reasons for this. First, some men think that a condom reduces their sexual pleasure. There is no way that this can be disproved or proved. Second, some men are embarrassed about buying condoms, although this reluctance might be becoming less common as condoms are available from vending machines.

If it's not on ...

Education about the use of condoms has increased the knowledge of their value, but has not changed young men's sexual behaviour in using them, according to a 1989 survey in the UK. To counter this lack of responsibility by some men, a number of female health professionals have suggested that sexually active teenage women buy and carry condoms with them. If a situation arises in which the young woman and man want to have sex, and he does not have a condom, she can produce one and say, 'Either you put this on, or there will be no sex. Think about it!' Or, as a recent advertisement said, 'If it's not on … it's not on!' A teenage woman has to be very self-assured to take this approach. For example, a woman might believe that if she insists the man use a condom and provides it, he will think she is a slut and will be turned off sexually. One young woman explained: 'It would be terrible if you were with this guy that you wanted to impress and you knock him rotten by saying, "Let's use this". And he looked at you as if you were some kind of a freak and turned on you and said, "Why, have you got something wrong with you?"'

Contraceptives for women

Women become pregnant, not men. Many men still believe that it is the woman's responsibility to prevent pregnancy, although this attitude is changing slowly. More men and women are talking to each other about contraceptive choices. But many are not.

Teenage women have several contraceptive choices, and the one most often chosen is the pill, although a few women choose the vaginal diaphragm. Some contraceptive methods that might be preferred by older women are not suitable for young women, especially if the woman has not had a child. An obvious example is sterilisation by tying the Fallopian tubes. The intrauterine device (IUD) (discussed later in this chapter) should not be a first choice of contraceptive for a teenage woman, although it could be chosen in certain circumstances, for example if the young woman cannot take the pill and neither she nor her male partner likes using condoms or a diaphragm. However, in this situation it is better not to use an IUD unless the woman and her partner are faithful to each other and neither has had previous sexual partners, as the risk of infection is higher.

The pill

Most sexually active young women who decide that they will use a contraceptive choose the pill. The pill is used by fifty-five million women around the world. It is chosen because it is very

Myths about the pill

- It is not true that the pill makes a woman promiscuous. People become 'sexual adventurers' for a number of reasons; taking the pill is not one of them.
- It is not true that the pill, if taken for a number of years, reduces a woman's chance of becoming pregnant when she stops. Most women who stop taking the pill in order to have a baby become pregnant within a year.
- It is not true that more deformed babies are born to women who have taken the pill.
- It is not true that if you take the pill for a number of years you are at greater risk of developing cancer. The pill reduces your chance of developing ovarian cancer or cancer of the lining of the uterus (endometrial cancer) in late middle age. The pill does not increase your chance of developing breast cancer.
- It is not true that taking the pill makes a woman depressed, although it can contribute to changes in mood, the most negative mood being during the week of inactive pills, when bleeding occurs. Depression is caused by a number of things; taking the pill is not one of them.
- It is not true that you cannot take the pill if you have varicose veins. The pill is not recommended only if you have varicose veins, are grossly overweight, and have had a clot in a deep vein.
- It is not true that the pill makes you put on weight, although your weight might fluctuate during the menstrual cycle.
- It is not true that you should stop taking the pill for a few months every two to three years, to give your body a rest. All this does is increase the chance that you will become pregnant because you are not taking the pill.

effective in preventing an unwanted pregnancy, it is safe for most women, and it is easy to take. One disadvantage for some teenage women is that it has to be prescribed by a doctor, which means that the teenager has to go to a private doctor or to a doctor at a family planning clinic to obtain it. Usually the doctor will ask the woman a few questions about past illnesses and check that she has normal blood pressure. The doctor will ask if she has had a vaginal examination before and if she has had a Pap smear taken. If she has not she or he will explain what is involved. If appropriate the doctor may suggest a vaginal examination and perhaps take a Pap smear (see chapter 4), if one hasn't been done in the previous year.

The pill contains hormones made in a laboratory that are similar to the hormones produced naturally in a woman's body. The pill prevents pregnancy in three ways. First, it prevents the development and release of an egg from the ovary. Second, it alters the nature of the lining of the uterus so that, if an egg is released, it would not be able to implant in the lining. Third, it thickens the secretions of the cervix so that sperm find it difficult to wiggle through to reach the cavity of the uterus and the Fallopian tube. This prevents the fertilisation of an egg by a sperm.

As well as protecting a woman against an unwanted pregnancy, the pill has other advantages. It reduces the severity of menstrual cramps, sometimes preventing them altogether. It regulates the menstrual periods and decreases the amount of menstrual flow. It reduces the chance that a woman will develop breast lumps. It improves acne in some young women. If a woman has several sexual partners (or her partner has had several sexual partners), the pill reduces the chance that she will be infected with a sexually transmitted disease, although in this respect it is not as effective as the use of a condom.

The pills available today contain a smaller amount of hormones compared with those prescribed twenty years ago, so that the reported side effects, such as vaginal candida infection, weight gain, and headaches, are now less likely to occur.

What the pill is like

Today's pills come in plastic packs, each tablet in a small bubble. Often the days are marked so that taking the pill is easier. There are two kinds of packs. In one the woman takes a tablet every day. This pack contains the pill in twenty-one bubbles and a sugar pill (sometimes an iron-containing pill) in the other

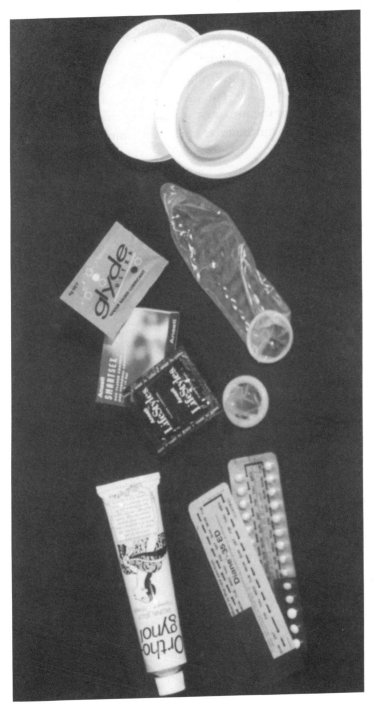

A range of contraceptive measures is available—the pill, spermicide, the condom, and the diaphragm.

seven. You can identify the inactive (sugar) pills because they are a different colour and there are only seven of them. This is the 'twenty-eight-day pill pack'. In the second formulation the pack contains twenty-one hormone pills. This is the 'twenty-one-day pill pack'. After the twenty-one days the woman has seven pill-free days. You can expect to have a period during the last seven days of pill-taking or when you are taking no tablets.

It does not matter which formulation you choose as long as you follow the instructions in the pack, but these are printed in tiny print and might seem intimidating. Because of this, a working party of manufacturers of the pill and medical experts in the USA have suggested that clearer instructions, written in simple English, would help a lot of pill users. Table 9.1 shows instructions modified from their paper and from other sources.

Table 9.1   How to take the pill

Please read these directions (and the manufacturer's directions if you have them) before you start taking the pill and any time you are not sure what to do.

The right way to take the pill is to take one pill every day at the same time.

If you miss any pills you may get pregnant, particularly if you start the pack late.

Before you start taking the pill
- Look at your pill pack to see if it has 28 or 21 pills.
- Find where on the pack you should start taking the pills.
- Find out in what order you should take the pills (follow the arrow).
- Be sure that you have another kind of contraceptive ready (such as condoms) to use as a back-up in case you miss any pills.
- Be sure that you always have a spare full pack of the pill.

When to start the first pack of pills
You have choices on which day you will start taking your first pack of pills. Decide with your doctor which is the best day for you.
- Pick a time of day that is easy to remember, and when you will always be able to take your pill.
- Check the manufacturer's instructions.

DAY 1 start: Take the active (coloured) pill of the first pack during the first 24 hours of your period, and continue for 21 days, then either have 7 days off or take 7 inactive pills.

SATURDAY start: Take the first active (coloured) pill of the first pack on the Saturday after your period starts, even if you are still bleeding.

If your period starts on Saturday, start the pack that day. But remember, you should use another contraceptive (such as a condom) as a back-up if you have sex at any time from the Saturday you start your first pack until the next Saturday (7 days later).

Whatever day you choose to start on, take one pill at the same time every day until the pack is finished. Don't skip pills, even if you are 'spotting' or bleeding between your periods.

During the first cycle you may feel a bit nauseated and may have little 'break through' bleeds. Both the nausea and the 'break through' bleeds cease after one or two cycles. If the bleeding is heavy, stop the pill and start a new pack on the usual day. If you are in any doubt, see your doctor.

When you finish the pack

- **21-day pill pack:** Wait 7 days to start the next pack. During this time you will probably have your period. Remember to make sure that no more than 7 days passes between 21-day packs.
- **28-day pill pack:** Start the next pack on the day after your last reminder pill. Do not miss any days between packs.

What to do if you miss a pill

1 If you MISS 1 active (coloured) pill and are less than 12 hours late
a) Take it as soon as you remember. Take your next pill at your regular time. This may mean that you take 2 pills in one day.
b) You do not need to use a back-up contraceptive if you have sex.

2 If you MISS 1 active pill and are more than 12 hours late
a) Take it as soon as you remember. Take your next pill at your regular time. This may mean that you take 2 pills in 1 day.
b) You should use back-up contraception if you have sex in the next 7 days.

3   If you MISS 2 active (coloured) pills in a row
a) Take 2 pills on the day you remember and 2 pills the next day.
b) After this continue with 1 pill every day till you finish the pack.
c) You may become pregnant if you have sex in the 7 days after you miss the pills. You must use another method of contraception (such as condoms) for the next 7 days.

What do you do if you miss a period?

* **If you have taken the pill correctly:** Don't worry. Continue with the new pack. If you miss two periods see your doctor or go to a family planning clinic.
* **If you miss one period and have missed taking your pill:** You need to have a pregnancy test done. Your can visit your pharmacist, doctor, or family planning doctor.

The minipill

This pill does not contain any oestrogen and is helpful for women who cannot take oestrogen. It is not as effective in preventing pregnancy as the combined oestrogen and progestogen pill. There are also longer acting implants (under the skin) and injections of progestogen available and suitable for some women. These can be discussed with a doctor.

Vaginal diaphragm

A vaginal diaphragm worn by a woman acts as a barrier. Vaginal diaphragms are made of a layer of latex attached to a circular latex rim. Different women's vaginas are of different sizes, so diaphragms are made in various sizes. Because of this the woman has to be examined, so that the doctor can determine the correct size. The woman has to learn to insert the diaphragm, to take it out, and to keep it clean. Learning is a little complicated, but once you have learnt to deal with a diaphragm it becomes easy.

The diaphragm has to be put into the vagina and correctly positioned before the couple have sex. After sex the diaphragm has to be left in the woman's vagina for eight to ten hours before it is taken out. It has to be washed and dried thoroughly before being returned to its box.

Teenage women do not often choose a diaphragm, unless they are in a permanent relationship, because of the problems of inserting, taking out, and storing the diaphragm. However, if the woman is familiar with her body, has learned to put in the diaphragm properly, and is motivated to use it, it places contraception under her control, which a condom does not.

Intrauterine device

The intrauterine device (IUD) is a plastic shape that can be placed inside the uterus (see figure 9.2). A doctor has to insert the IUD after examining the woman. Once it is inside, the IUD usually remains there, preventing pregnancy by altering the nature of the lining of the uterus. It could be uncomfortable or painful having an IUD inserted, and crampy pains sometimes persist for two or three days. If they persist for more than seven days, the woman should see her doctor. Some women have slight spotting or bleeding for one or two months after the insertion.

The IUD has a string that projects through the cervix into the vagina. As a woman's uterus sometimes expels the IUD, usually during menstruation, a woman should return to her doctor after the first period following the insertion to make

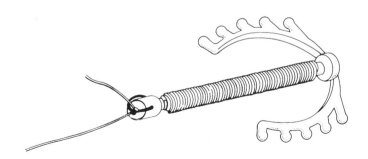

Figure 9.2 The IUD, much enlarged in size.

sure that everything is in order. She should also feel for the string inside her vagina after every period, and if she can't find it, visit a doctor.

A woman who has not had children and who has or has had several sexual partners, or whose partner has had several sexual partners, should not choose an IUD. The reason is that she might have been infected with *Chlamydia* during sexual intercourse and the organism could lurk in the cells lining her cervical canal without causing any symptoms. If she has an IUD inserted, some of the organisms could be carried up into her uterus and cause pelvic inflammatory disease (PID). PID causes an offensive vaginal discharge and lower abdominal pain. If the organisms were carried into the uterus by the IUD, these symptoms will occur within twenty days of the IUD insertion. If the symptoms occur after that time, the infection was not carried into the uterus by the IUD, but has occurred following sex with an infected partner, whose sperm carried the *Chlamydia* from the cervix into the uterus. Studies show that about one sexually active woman in every thousand will develop PID each year. Nearly all these women have several sexual partners (or their partner has or has had several sexual partners) and are younger than 25. Fewer than 1 per cent of these women have used an IUD. PID is discussed further in chapter 12.

Health care

- Check for the string several times in the first month and at least following your period each month thereafter. If you can't feel the string, visit your doctor.
- If you develop fever, pain in your pelvis, bad cramps, or smelly vaginal discharge, or if you experience pain when you have intercourse, see your doctor immediately. These symptoms might be signs of a sexually transmitted infection that needs treatment.
- If you miss a menstrual period see your doctor or family planning clinic.

Periodic abstinence

In this method a woman learns to recognise the changes in the wetness of her vagina that occur during the menstrual cycle (see figure 9.3). As ovulation time approaches the secretions of the cervix increase and the nature of the secretions changes. They become less sticky and clearer. A woman might 'feel' the change, but usually needs to insert a finger into her vagina or place a tissue at its entrance to detect changes. After ovulation the secretions change again and become sticky and decrease in amount. The woman learns not to have sexual intercourse when the watery secretion is present, especially when it is profuse and clear in texture. Learning how to recognise changes in the secretions is complicated, and is taught in classes by 'natural family planning associations'. Most teenagers are unwilling to attend such classes as they are usually run for married couples.

The 'morning-after' pill

This is an emergency method of preventing an unwanted pregnancy. If a woman has sexual intercourse at about ovulation time (see above) and neither she nor the man is using contraceptives, she has a 30 per cent chance of becoming pregnant. If she doesn't want to become pregnant she could choose the 'morning-after' pill, which is a high-dose hormonal progestogen-only pill. She does not have to take the medication the morning after, but must obtain the tablets from a doctor or a family planning clinic within seventy-two hours of having unprotected intercourse. She takes two progestogen pills at once and two more progestogen pills twelve hours later. Nausea is seldom a problem with the current morning-after pills. The morning-after pill works by altering the lining of the uterus so that the egg cannot implant in it.

Because the morning-after pill is not always effective, it should not be used as a regular method of birth control, but should be kept for a real emergency. When it is taken because of

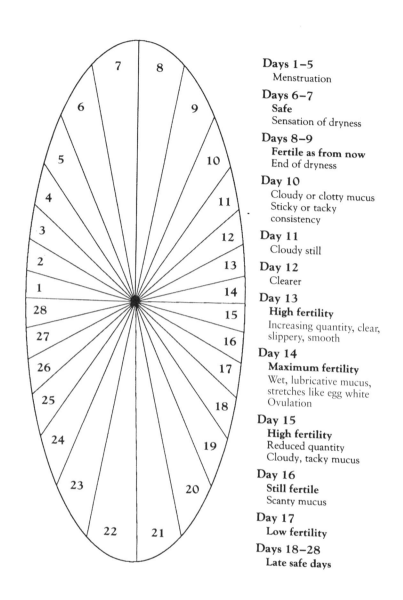

Days 1–5
Menstruation

Days 6–7
Safe
Sensation of dryness

Days 8–9
Fertile as from now
End of dryness

Day 10
Cloudy or clotty mucus
Sticky or tacky
consistency

Day 11
Cloudy still

Day 12
Clearer

Day 13
High fertility
Increasing quantity, clear,
slippery, smooth

Day 14
Maximum fertility
Wet, lubricative mucus,
stretches like egg white
Ovulation

Day 15
High fertility
Reduced quantity
Cloudy, tacky mucus

Day 16
Still fertile
Scanty mucus

Day 17
Low fertility

Days 18–28
Late safe days

Figure 9.3 Changes in fertility and in vaginal secretions over the menstrual cycle. These changes are monitored by women using periodic abstinence as a method of contraception.

unprotected intercourse at ovulation time, it prevents pregnancy nine times out of ten. But if the woman does not have a period at the expected time, she should consult a doctor and have a pregnancy test.

Myths about contraception

Since contraception has not been openly discussed until recently, it is not surprising that there are many myths about it.

- 'If you have sex standing up, you won't get pregnant.' If you have sex when you are ovulating (that is, in the middle part of the cycle between your periods), you probably will become pregnant, regardless of the position you were in during intercourse.
- 'I don't need contraception because pregnancy can't happen to me.' It can!
- 'Douching is an effective way of preventing pregnancy.' It isn't! It is like shutting the stable door when the horse is inside.
- 'If you urinate as soon as the man has "come" inside you, you won't get pregnant.' You can!

Failure rates of contraception among teenagers

Not all contraceptive methods are equally effective in preventing pregnancy. In some cases the failure of the contraceptive is because the person does not use the contraceptive method properly or takes a chance and from time to time does not use it at all. The use of condoms is an example. As mentioned earlier, some young men dislike wearing condoms. A man might suggest to his partner that, as she is not near the time when she is expected to be ovulating, he doesn't need to wear a condom.

In other cases, the failure to prevent pregnancy is due to the method itself. The failure rate is defined in the following way: of 100 teenagers who use the method for one year, the number who become pregnant is [x].

The failure rate of the available contraceptive methods is shown in table 9.1.

Table 9.1 The yearly failure rate of contraceptives (in terms of resultant pregnancies) among teenagers

Contraceptive	%
Pill	0.25
Minipill	2
IUD	2.5
Condom	5
Diaphragm	10
Spermicidal foams	15
Periodic abstinence	20
Withdrawal	25
Chance	90

Chapter Ten

Teenage pregnancy

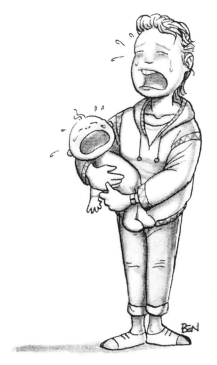

Experience is the name everyone gives to their mistakes.

Oscar Wilde, Lady Windermere's Fan

One of the consequences of sexual intercourse, if contraceptives are not used, is that the woman might become pregnant. Unfortunately, 25 per cent or more of sexually active teenagers do not use contraceptives, at least in the first months after starting intercourse. The younger the woman, the less likely she is to be taking the pill, and the younger the man, the less likely he is to be using a condom. In most countries, the teenage male believes it is the woman's responsibility to use contraceptives. In any month, if a woman has sex at ovulation time and neither she nor her partner uses contraceptives, she has a one in three chance of becoming pregnant. Of course, if she knew that pregnancy is only likely to occur on the days around ovulation, and if she avoided sexual intercourse at the time, pregnancy would be unlikely to occur.

It appears that few teenage women know when ovulation occurs during the menstrual cycle. In one survey, we found that six out of ten teenage women had no idea when ovulation occurred, and the same number were unaware that pregnancy is most likely to occur if a couple have sex during the time around ovulation.

These two factors—lack of contraceptive use and ignorance about when ovulation occurs—increase the chance of a sexually active teenage woman becoming pregnant. And a large number of teenage women do. Studies in the United States, the UK, and Australia show that in any year one of every ten to twenty teenage women becomes pregnant, and more than 90 per cent of these teenagers are unmarried at the time. In the United States in 1996, there were about ten million teenage women, and 47 per cent of them were sexually active. This meant that nearly five million teenage women were at risk of becoming pregnant; and nearly a million (950,000) did.

In Australia in 1996, there were more than 600,000 teenage women, and one in forty of them became pregnant. We do not know exactly how many Australian teenagers have sexual intercourse, but surveys made in 1996 suggest that by the age of 16, 21 per cent of girls had had sexual intercourse at least once, and by the age of 19, more than 50 per cent of teenage women had had sex at least once. Similar figures are reported from a survey made in the UK. The survey showed that by the age of 16, 35 per cent of boys and 25 per cent of girls had had sexual intercourse at least once.

The good news is that in all three countries the number of teenage pregnancies is falling, particularly in some parts of the USA and UK. This is not because of an increased number of abortions, but because more young women are using contraceptives. The question teenagers and adults should be asking is: Can the number of unexpected, unintended pregnancies be reduced? It can. A study made by the Guttmacher Institute of adolescent sexual behaviour and pregnancy in Canada, the UK, France, the Netherlands, and Sweden found that:

- Fewer adolescents become pregnant if they have had good sex education.
- Fewer adolescents become pregnant in countries where contraceptive advice is readily available. The United States has recently reduced its high adolescent birth rates by improving education programs about contraception.
- Teenagers are not too immature to use contraceptives effectively.
- In countries studied, the low adolescent birth rates (compared with the United States and some other countries) were not achieved by the teenagers having abortions.
- More socially deprived, poverty-stricken teenagers, from dysfunctional families, are likely to have sex and become pregnant than are girls from better-off families. Poverty is a major factor, which also affects the other factors listed.
- Welfare benefits (single parent pension) and services do not act as an inducement to teenagers to have babies.

It should be noted that in most cases of adolescent pregnancy the man involved is older than the teenage girl, and is often an adult. He is therefore more likely to be sexually experienced, possibly to have a sexually transmitted disease, and to have greater power to persuade the girl to agree to sexual intercourse.

Choices

When a teenage woman discovers that she is pregnant she has several choices:

- She and the father of the unborn child talk it over and might decide to marry or live together and share childcare.
- Her parents, on hearing her news, put pressure on her and the man to make them marry. This might be traumatic, and she might seek counselling.
- She decides that she does not want to marry the child's father and might choose to have the baby 'out of wedlock' with or without his support. If she makes this choice she will have to decide whether she wants to keep the baby (most women do) and be an 'unmarried mother'. Unmarried mothers encountered difficulties in housing and in financial support, but with better, more humane social attitudes since the 1980s, these difficulties have been reduced considerably. On the other hand, she might choose to have her baby adopted.
- She decides after talking with a counsellor (and her parents) that she will have an abortion. If her parents agree with this decision, she will receive their support in the weeks after the abortion, which can be an emotional time. If, on the other hand, her parents forbid her from having an abortion, in spite of her wishes, the family might need to seek the help of a counsellor. Ultimately, the pregnant woman's decision is paramount. This also applies if her parents try to insist that she has an abortion and she does not want to destroy her child.

It can be difficult for a pregnant teenager to decide what she thinks is best for her, and often professional counselling will help her. If she has a close relationship with her parents she will be able to talk about the choices with them; but if she and they have difficulty in talking to each other, an experienced counsellor can help them explore their feelings about the pregnancy and help them to reach a decision. In the end, however, the teenager has to make a choice with which she is comfortable.

Which choices do pregnant teenagers make?

Studies from the four countries shown in figure 10.1 show a remarkable similarity of choice.

- Between 20 and 30 per cent of unmarried, pregnant teenagers choose to have the baby and are married by the time the baby is born.
- Between 20 and 30 per cent of the unmarried teenagers choose to have the baby 'out of wedlock'. Most keep and rear the baby; a few give up the baby for adoption.
- Between 45 and 50 per cent of pregnant, teenage women choose to have an abortion.

Perceptions of pregnancy and parenting

Studies in several countries show that the expectations pregnant, teenage girls have of the pregnancy and parenting are not always correct. A few young women avoid using contraceptives and become pregnant in the belief that pregnancy will be happiest time of their life. For some young women this belief and the reality match; for others pregnancy is not as pleasant as they had anticipated. Some young women also believe that having a baby will solve their problems of being bored, lonely, and dissatisfied with life. Once again the reality might be different, if the woman finds that her baby is constantly demanding.

Medical consequences of teenage pregnancy

The medical literature suggests that pregnancy causes more problems if a woman is teenaged and particularly if she is aged 16 or younger. The reports suggest that young, teenage, pregnant women have a greater chance of giving birth to a low birth-weight (so-called premature) baby, and have a greater chance of developing anaemia or a raised blood pressure in pregnancy. More recent reports show that these complications

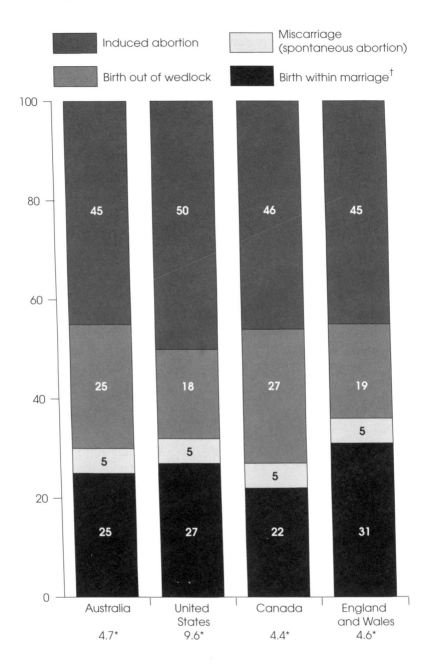

Figure 10.1 Women younger than 20 who became pregnant during 1986–96.
†Half conceived outside marriage. *Percentage pregnant each year.

are less likely to occur if the teenager attends a doctor or a clinic early in the pregnancy, preferably in the first ten weeks. They are less likely to occur if she has a professional person with whom she can talk and who gives her advice about her diet (which she follows), and if she stops or reduces cigarette smoking and alcohol intake and avoids other habit-forming drugs. Teenage women are no more likely to have a difficult childbirth than women aged 20–29.

Social consequences of teenage motherhood

Whether or not the teenage mother is married she faces several social problems. The pregnancy and the need to care for the baby mean that usually she has to give up work, training for work, or schooling. By the time the child is old enough to go to childcare, the mother might not want to start training again and, if she chooses to work, can often only obtain a poorly paid job with few prospects.

It is also known that marriages between teenagers are likely to break down, especially when they occur either following or because of a pregnancy. The divorce rate for women who married when they were teenagers is twice that of women who married when they were in their twenties, and after seven years, three couples in five who married as teenagers will have divorced. The divorce occurs at a time when the child is particularly vulnerable to the effects of the changes that have occurred.

If the teenage woman chooses to be an unmarried mother, the effects of motherhood on her opportunity to train or to continue her education might be even greater than if she were married. If her parents are supportive the negative effects are reduced, but if her parents reject her or behave coldly to her, she might become depressed and even need psychiatric care. Alternatively, she might form a new relationship, which might lead to the same consequence as the first. The social consequences will vary to some extent, depending on the young woman's expectations. Some teenage mothers do not want to follow a career or obtain further training. They live from day to day, and the baby does not interrupt their life to any major degree. Others have a romantic image of motherhood that fails to be realised when the woman has to face the reality of caring for a baby who is demanding, unpredictable, and exhausting. The young mother might become depressed and unable to cope unless she has strong family support.

Of course, these bad results affect a minority of unmarried teenage mothers. Many form a new relationship in which the woman is loved, loves her partner, and is happy.

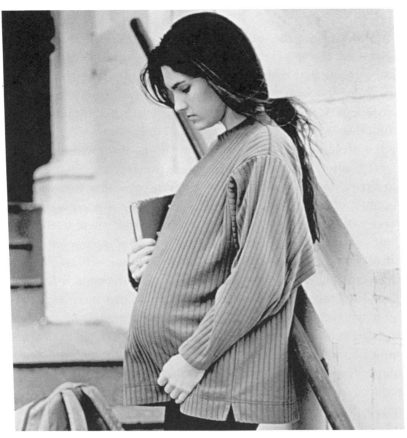

Teenage motherhood—some young women cope very well with the lifestyle changes motherhood brings, and others have problems, especially if they lack family support.

Abortion

Contrary to popular belief, the choice of abortion is not an easy one, and most teenagers think long and deeply before they decide. Provided the abortion is performed by a qualified person in a well-equipped hospital or clinic, the procedure involves only slight danger. Only one woman in every thousand either develops a fever lasting more than three days (requiring antibiotics) or has continued bleeding from the uterus (requiring injections or further surgery).

The problems of having an abortion performed are reduced still further if the operation is done before the pregnancy has reached twelve weeks (dated from the first day of the last period). The operation will be performed after injecting an anaesthetic into the cervix or, less commonly, after giving a general anaesthetic. The fetus, in its sac, and the placenta are sucked out of the uterus through a soft plastic tube. The operation takes about five minutes.

Afterwards, the woman remains in the hospital or clinic for about two hours, and regular observations are made by the staff. The observations are to check the amount of bleeding that occurs, the pulse rate, and blood pressure. During this time the staff talk with the teenager and answer her questions. She is usually given antibiotics to take and is asked to report if she develops a fever or if the bleeding from her vagina becomes heavy. Bleeding usually lasts for five or six days and is like a heavy period. Some women have little or no bleeding; some might bleed for two weeks. Often there is little bleeding for the first two days, and then a fair amount occurs in the next three to six days. Some women experience uterine cramps for several days. These usually respond to Naprogesic or to Ponstan.

It is important that a woman who has had an abortion be examined about two weeks after the operation. The purpose of the examination is to make sure that the uterus has returned to its non-pregnant size and that there is no infection in the pelvis. The opportunity is taken to talk more about family planning (contraception), which was discussed just before the abortion was performed. Even more importantly, the teenager might want to talk about her feelings regarding the abortion and have questions she wants answered.

Following an abortion a woman could have one or more fears. The first is that she will be unable to become pregnant later. The second is that if she does become pregnant, the baby will be born early and will not be healthy. The third is that she will become pregnant again. In most abortion services the teenager is given the opportunity to talk with a trained counsellor. The counsellor will be able to reassure her that her fears are unfounded. An abortion, performed as we have described, is extremely unlikely to prevent a future pregnancy, nor is any future baby likely to be born early or damaged.

Ethical problems of abortion

Abortion is a sensitive subject and arouses strong emotions among adults and teenagers. Some people believe that abortion is an evil and should never (or hardly ever) be allowed. These people believe that human life begins the moment the sperm penetrates the egg. If any attempt is made to interrupt the pregnancy, it is like murdering the embryo or the fetus. To these people, abortion should never be contemplated, even in the case of rape or incest or if the fetus is severely deformed.

Other people believe that the embryo and the fetus, at least in the first twenty weeks of pregnancy, is not a human being but a potential human being. It is only a potential human being because it is incapable of surviving outside its mother's uterus. These people believe that in the early part of pregnancy the mother has the right to decide what she wants to do about the pregnancy.

The people who support relaxation of laws against abortion point out that even in countries where there are strict laws against abortion, women obtain them anyway. Rich women either go to another country where abortion laws are less strict, or pay large sums of money to have an abortion performed by a doctor. Poor women do not have these choices. If a poor woman decides to have an abortion because of family circumstances, or the anxiety that another baby will jeopardise the survival of her existing children, or for many other reasons, she has to go to a 'backyard abortionist'. Although some backyard abortionists are skilled, many are dangerous and dirty. Although the woman obtains an abortion, she might become infected or even bleed to death. If infection occurs—as often happens—she can become very ill and possibly even sterile. People who support relaxation of the laws prohibiting abortion say that in countries where legal abortion is permitted, the sad and serious consequences of backyard abortions are eliminated. Women who choose to have an abortion in these countries know that it will be done safely by a trained health professional.

The debate will continue, but whatever the laws, women will continue to end unwanted, unwelcomed pregnancies by seeking an abortion. The only way for abortions to be reduced in frequency is for all couples to be able to obtain contraceptives easily.

Chapter Eleven

Sexual abuse

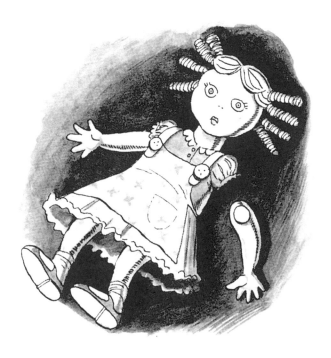

Sexual assault is not about sex. It is about power relationships between people. Sexual assault is a violation of basic human rights ...

Pamphlet

Sexual abuse—including rape and incest—occurs when another person touches or fondles a part of the body that has sexual attributes, according to the belief of the society in which the person lives. In Western societies these areas include the female breasts and the genital and anal areas of both sexes. In some cases sexual abuse can be said to have occurred if a person is kissed against his or her will. Sexual harassment occurs when a person makes insulting or derogatory remarks or is overtly sexual (for example, flashing his penis) to another person who is usually of the opposite sex.

Studies in Australasia, the UK, and the USA suggest that between 10 and 25 per cent of female children and adolescents younger than 16 have been sexually abused, and rather more have been physically abused. In half the reported cases, the girl's breasts or genitals were touched, and in 5 to 10 per cent, the girl's abuser had attempted or had succeeded in having vaginal or anal intercourse. The abuser was a family member (including a stepfather and de facto father) in nearly half of all cases of sexual abuse. If the abuser was the girl's father, stepfather, or de facto father, in 75 per cent of cases he was also in an abusive relationship with the girl's mother.

Studies in the countries mentioned indicate that sexually abused women, compared with females who have not been sexually abused:

- are two to five times as likely to have low self-esteem
- are two to four times more likely to suicide
- are two to three times as likely to have psychological, psychiatric, or sexual problems when adults
- are more likely to develop an eating disorder or to have disordered eating
- are twice as likely to divorce if they marry.

Whether these findings are applicable to women in other countries is not known.

In the case of a young woman, the sexual abuser is usually her father; less often it is an uncle, a grandfather, a brother, or stepfather. Usually the girl is the first born or the only girl in the family. In many cases the abuse begins when she is as young as

4 or 5 years old. The man might entice the girl to sit on his knee and persuade her to fondle his penis or to suck it. To encourage her, he might show her pornographic pictures or talk to her provocatively. He might fondle her genitals and, in some cases, force her to have sexual intercourse when she is as young as 8 years old. And this pattern might continue until the girl is in her teens or reports the abuse. Many of the abusers demand absolute obedience from all family members and rule the family by violent behaviour. Many are heavy drinkers.

Even if the girl wants to resist she can't, because she will be threatened or beaten. If she talks to her mother, she is likely to find that her mother doesn't believe her and sides with her father or the male being questioned. Some mothers might be so frightened of the man that they do not interfere, even when they know that their daughters are being sexually abused. Incest is hidden deep in the family, and when the girl and her abuser are together outside the family, they appear to have a normal relationship.

It is important to remember that when sexual abuse occurs it is not the fault of the person being abused nor is it the fault of the person's mother.

Effects of sexual abuse

The effects of sexual abuse can be considerable. If the female is a young girl or a teenager she might do poorly at school. She might daydream and be withdrawn, or she might act up, seeking attention. Often she finds it difficult to develop a close relationship with another girl or another teenager. As she reaches late adolescence and becomes an adult she might have sexual problems. She might be repelled by sexual intercourse or submit but not enjoy sex, because of her experiences when she was younger. She might be disturbed psychologically, being depressed or anxious and unable to relate to anyone. If she feels that she is able to talk openly to someone about the abuse, she might benefit from counselling, which might be needed for a long period of time.

On the other hand, there is evidence that many, perhaps most, young women cope well and become well-adjusted adults and fully functioning lovers and parents. It is untrue that all women (and men) who were sexually abused in childhood will become abusing parents. Some will, others will not.

The chance of problems developing following sexual abuse can be reduced considerably if the young woman does not keep the abuse secret but seeks help and support as early as she can. There are dangers, however, if the young woman does not follow this advice—because she is afraid or insecure or does not know who to tell—that she will keep the matter secret until she has become an adult. Then, if she is unhappy or has psychological problems, she might seek the help of a psychologist or a psychiatrist.

Some psychological counsellors believe that a wide variety of psychological problems experienced by adult women can be traced back to childhood sexual abuse. These problems include personality disorders, relationship problems, sexual problems, and eating disorders. In some instances her therapist is correct and, when the woman feels that she can trust the therapist, she will admit that she was sexually abused, and the healing process can start.

But if the woman continues to deny that she was sexually abused, a few psychologists believe that the woman has suppressed all the memory of the assault and that she has the 'suppressed memory syndrome'. The psychologist then persuades the woman that if she accepts and believes that she was sexually abused, usually by a parent or close relative, her current problems will be cured. The consequences of this fantasy can be detrimental to the woman, not helpful. She becomes distrustful of everyone, thus aggravating her problem. The 'knowledge' might destroy her relationship with her parents and close family. It might lead to unjustified legal proceedings against a parent or a relative.

A few women are so traumatised by sexual abuse in childhood that they suppress the memory, but the vast majority of sexually assaulted women (and men) remember the event or repeated events only too clearly.

Help for victims of sexual abuse

Feeling supported and believed by their mother, after she has been told of the abuse, is the most important factor in recovery. A major problem is that many people do not believe children and young teenagers when they say that they have been sexually assaulted by a family member. Children and young teenagers who say they have been sexually assaulted should always be believed. This is particularly true of young children who tell of sexual interference. They rarely, if ever, make the story up, simply because they usually do not have the knowledge or the experience to imagine such a story. If older people believe a young person when she complains of sexual abuse, it would help to reduce the frequency of that abuse.

Reducing the incidence of sexual abuse

Reducing the incidence of sexual abuse is difficult as in most cases the abuser has so much power over the victim that she (or he) is afraid of telling anyone about the abuse. The young girl may not realise abuse is wrong or she may feel responsible and blame herself. The situation is improving as sexual abuse is talked about more openly and society acknowledges it is a serious problem. Information is being made available in schools, so that a child or a teenager *can* feel that they can tell other people if they have been sexually interfered with or assaulted. And they should be made aware that if they are not believed the first time, they should tell the story again, and they should go on telling it until someone helps them.

One practical way in which children can be helped to avoid incest is to teach them, from the time that they are toddlers, about 'good touching' and 'bad touching'. Children should be taught that some parts of their bodies are not available to be touched and certain forms of behaviour are not appropriate, even if the person who wants to engage in this form of behaviour is a parent, a relative, or a close friend.

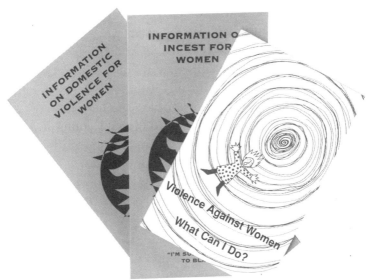

Many brochures and information leaflets explain to victims of rape and incest the counselling options available and what they can expect if they plan to press charges, and generally offer much-needed support.

This message about 'good' or 'bad' touching can be changed as the child grows older and starts to have relationships outside the family, so that they can develop a normal sexual relationship.

Rape

Rape occurs when one person forces another to have sexual intercourse (which includes oral and anal sex); at the time of the assault, the person is forced against their will. Usually, the rapist is a man and the person raped is a woman, but in some circumstances, in gaols for example, rape of males by males is not unusual.

In cases of male–female rape, the woman will be forced to have sexual intercourse, or to suck the man's penis until he ejaculates in her mouth, or to submit to anal intercourse. Sometimes the man inserts a bottle or a stick into her vagina or anus. If the woman is assaulted by a gang of men (a 'gang bang') she will be subjected to these sorts of attacks with each man or simultaneously by more than one man. A rapist has a contempt for women. He treats the woman as an object, not as a person. Society lets men believe that they are sexual predators or that they are sex experts. Society lets men believe that most women really want sex but are too shy to ask. A rapist sees himself as a tiger or a wolf and his victim as his prey—a chicken, a bird, or a lamb. Many rapists are insecure in their relationships with other people. They are excited by causing pain. They are stimulated by the feeling of power and by being able to humiliate the woman. One rapist has said: 'I despise a woman who gives in to men; and hate her if she doesn't.'

Myths about rape

MYTH   Nearly all rapists are strangers.

FACT   Most rapists are well-known to the victim. Often the man is a member of her family or a close family friend.

MYTH   Rapists are violent, sick, crazy men.

FACT   Most rapists look and act like ordinary men. They might be 'sick', but usually they are not mentally disturbed.

MYTH   Women ask to be raped because of their behaviour or because they dress provocatively.

FACT   No woman asks to be raped. Rape is a brutal, degrading experience. A woman's behaviour or the way she dresses does not lead to rape.

MYTH   Rapes occur because men can't control their sexual urges.

FACT   Most rapes are premeditated and planned. Men can control their sexual urges if they want to.

MYTH   Men rape women to obtain sexual relief.

FACT   Men rape women to dominate, to humiliate, and to show their contempt for and hatred of women.

MYTH   Most rapists are working-class, foreign-born men.

FACT   Rapists come from all classes of society, all ethnic groups, all religions.

MYTH   A woman can't be raped by her husband.

FACT   A woman who is forced against her will to submit to sexual assault by her husband is being raped.

There are many myths about rape; some of them are listed on p. 194.

Effects of rape

Rape is a humiliating, a degrading, and sometimes a terrifying experience. A rapist might bruise or scratch his victim, or hurt her genitals or her mouth. Even if she has no physical damage, she is usually, but not always, hurt emotionally.

Women cope with being raped in many different ways. Some women feel dirty. Some women feel ashamed. Some women become depressed, cry a lot, are unable to sleep, or just feel numb. Nothing matters any more. Some women cope by trying to forget the rape, by eliminating the rape from their thoughts; others want to talk incessantly about the rape. If the disturbing, negative feelings (shame, depression, feeling dirty) persist over a period of time, the woman might feel that she is going crazy, that she has a sexually transmitted disease, or that she will never get over the rape.

Women do get over rape. Recovery from the effects of being raped is quicker and easier if, as soon as possible after the rape, you can have someone you can talk to: someone you like and respect, someone who will be supportive, who believes your story, and who treats you as a human being. Remember, rape is *never* the woman's fault.

What should you do if you are raped?

If you have been raped you need help and support. You might get this from your family, or you might seek help from a sexual assault centre, a rape crisis centre, or a hospital. If you can, contact someone in your family or a friend you can trust. Ask the person to stay with you if you decide to go to hospital or report the rape to the police.

Do not wash, shower, have a bath, or change your clothes before going to the centre, the hospital, or the police. If you do you might destroy evidence that will be needed if there is a court case. Don't drink any alcohol in case it is claimed that you were drunk and encouraged the rapist.

If you decide to report the rape to the police, they will ask you to tell them what happened so that they can catch the person who raped you. If you wish, you can make a formal statement, in which case the police can bring the case to court.

This is what you do if you choose to make a formal statement:

- The statement has to be taken down in writing, and you will be asked to sign it.

- If you wish, you can ask for a female police officer to take the statement.

- It often takes a long time to make the statement, and you can have someone you know with you. If you want to rest for a while when you are making the statement, you may do so. Most police officers are very supportive.

- You will have to be examined by a doctor at a hospital. The examination includes the doctor asking you to tell your story once again. Then the doctor will examine you, noting bruises, scratches, and so on. The doctor will want to examine you vaginally and will take swabs from your vulva and from your vagina. All the medical evidence taken from you, including the swabs, is confidential and will not be disclosed to anyone but you for about three days. This is to let you make up your mind whether you want to go on with the police case. If you don't, the legal matters end there; but you should visit the doctor again so that you can learn whether you have been infected with a sexually transmitted disease or if you are worried you might be pregnant, and so you can talk with the doctor about your feelings if you wish.

In trying to decide whether you want to prosecute, you might want to talk with someone else, perhaps a counsellor at a rape crisis centre, or a social worker or a psychologist. You have to decide what is best for you.

Chapter Twelve

Sexually transmitted diseases

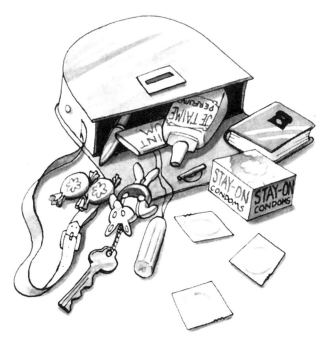

An ounce of prevention is worth a pound
of cure.

Proverb

One of the consequences of having sexual intercourse (particularly if you have sex with more than one person) is that you might become infected during sex with an illness that is transferred from one person to another. In other words, you could acquire a sexually transmitted disease (STD). Figures from several countries, especially the United States, show that infections which are always, or usually, transmitted during sexual intercourse are increasing among younger women. The more sexual partners a teenage woman has, the more likely she is to catch one of the sexually transmitted diseases. But you only need to have sex once with an infected man to have a high chance of being infected. Some of the sexually transmitted diseases are listed in this chapter. Two other diseases that are often sexually transmitted, *Candida* and trichomoniasis, cause a vaginal discharge and are described in chapter 14.

Non-gonococcal genital infection

Non-gonococcal genital infection (NGGI) is a name given to a group of bacteria that cause an infection of the internal pelvic organs. The most important of the organisms is called *Chlamydia*, and it accounts for more than half of all non-gonococcal genital infections. Until recently it was difficult to diagnose *Chlamydia*. Now a special pathology test has been developed which can detect *Chlamydia* in women's urine or in a sample taken by swab or brush from the woman's cervix.

This test has shown that between 1 and 10 per cent of sexually active young women are found to have chlamydial infection of the cells lining the cervical canal; and blood tests show that about one sexually active woman in every three younger than 30 has evidence of past infection. The chance of being infected increases if the woman has had sex with several partners or if her sexual partner has had sex with several women. Unless you are sure about your partner's sexual behaviour, it is wise to insist that he may not have sex with you unless he uses a condom.

In men, chlamydial infection (known as non-gonococcal ure-thritis) is a relatively mild condition. In women, chlamydial infection can cause serious problems if it is not detected and treated soon after infection occurs. All too often chlamydial infection is not detected because there are no symptoms. The woman does not know that she has been infected, but she can infect her sexual partner. Usually the infection is confined to her cervix, as mentioned earlier. Only if the infection affects the other genital organs, spreading through her uterus and infecting the Fallopian tubes, do symptoms occur, and even then there are often no symptoms (see figure 12.1). The symptoms of pelvic inflammatory disease (PID) are lower abdominal pain, an offen-sive-smelling vaginal discharge, and a fever. If PID is diagnosed, treatment is relatively easy. The woman (and any sexual part-ners) takes antibiotics for ten days.

If the woman has no symptoms and is not treated, she might find out that she was previously infected only if she has diffi-culty becoming pregnant. Investigations performed to discover

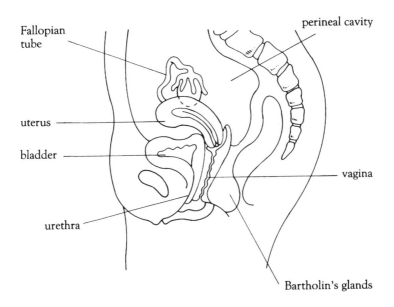

Figure 12.1 Where non-gonococcal genital infection attacks.

the cause of infertility might reveal that she has blocked Fallopian tubes, a sign of previous chlamydial infection.

Of course, not all women infected with *Chlamydia* develop PID. After one attack about 15 per cent of infected women will have damaged Fallopian tubes. If the woman has a second infection, the risk increases to 30 per cent, and after three infections the risk increases to 60 per cent.

There are three ways of avoiding chlamydial infection. The first is to avoid having sex. The second is to be absolutely sure that your partner has not had sex with any other person. The third way is to insist that your partner wear a condom if you can't trust him to tell the truth and if you are not sure of his previous sexual behaviour.

Genital warts

Tiny little areas of cauliflower warts appear on a woman's vulva or, less commonly, in her vagina, weeks or months after having intercourse with an infected man (see figure 12.2).

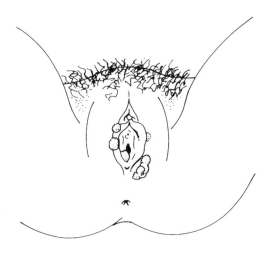

Figure 12.2 Genital warts on the vulva.

The warts are caused by a virus. If a woman finds she has warts, she should see a doctor to be treated, as the wart virus might be involved in causing cancer of the cervix (cervical cancer) years later. Treatment is to paint the warts with a substance called podophyllin or to use one of the newer agents that change the immune system or to freeze them with nitrous oxide. All these treatments are done in the doctor's office, and are usually not painful.

Following treatment the woman must have a Pap smear every six months and the vulva needs to be examined using a microscope (colposcopy) to see if there is any evidence of the virus, which is called HPV or Human Papilloma Virus.

Genital herpes

The virus that causes genital herpes is the cousin of the herpes virus that causes coldsores on the lips and the virus that causes chicken pox. If the woman has sexual intercourse with a man who has herpes blisters on his penis she is likely to be infected.

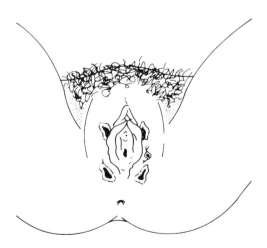

Figure 12.3 Genital herpes on a woman's vulva.

Five to ten days later, small areas that burn and itch appear on her labia. The next day reddish bumps appear that form small blisters (see figure 12.3). Sometimes the woman's whole vulva becomes swollen and painful. The blisters turn into very painful ulcers, which 'crust over' and heal in about five to seven days. During this time the woman is infectious because the ulcers shed large amounts of virus. Because of this the woman should wear pants at all times, in case she scratches the ulcers during sleep and transfers the virus to her mouth or eyes.

The virus tracks down the nerves that supply the area, and forms nests in a swollen part of the nerve near the spinal cord. The herpes virus might live quietly in the nerve and cause no further trouble. But in 50 per cent of women it tracks back along the nerve to form a new crop of blisters and ulcers. This can occur at any time but seems to occur more frequently after stress or another infection, or if the woman is 'run down'. Luckily most women have only one further attack, but a few have repeated attacks of herpes. Sometimes, an attack occurs every month, usually in the days before menstruation, or even more often.

Drugs called Acyclovir, Valacyclovir and Famivir are available for women who have regular attacks of herpes. The drugs are taken each day and reduce the number of recurrences from more than ten per year to less than two. These drugs can also be taken intermittently, if the attacks are less frequent and of decreasing severity. Trying to be in good health and, if possible, not stressed will help the frequency and severity of the attacks.

Genital herpes has another sinister effect. If a woman develops a first attack of genital herpes, or has a recurrence, in late pregnancy, the baby might be affected during childbirth. Doctors are aware of this and test these women each week in the last two to four weeks of pregnancy.

Gonorrhoea

Gonorrhoea affects about one sexually active teenage woman in every 500. The more sexual partners the woman has, the more likely she is to be infected. The *Gonococcus* is a delicate germ. It dies when dried or exposed to sunshine, which means you can't catch gonorrhoea from a toilet seat. It is caught by having sexual intercourse with an infected man.

In the body, the germ that causes gonorrhoea invades the tissues of the urethra and the cervix. Most men infected with gonorrhoea develop a purulent discharge from the urethra and have severe pain on urination. Most women have no symptoms. But if they have been infected they can infect their next sexual partner, or the germ might infect their Fallopian tubes and cause sterility (see figure 12.4). Because of this, women who have several sexual partners would be wise to have checks made by a doctor every six months.

Gonorrhoea is easily diagnosed and treated with antibiotics. Usually a single big dose of a penicillin is given. The woman takes the tablets by mouth, and takes a second kind of tablet at the same time and again six to twelve hours later. This second tablet acts to keep a high level of penicillin in the blood so that all the gonococci are killed. Nowadays, because women infected

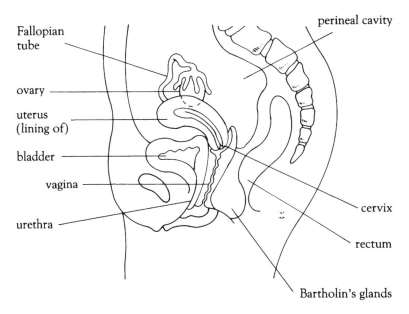

Figure 12.4 Where gonorrhoea attacks.

with gonorrhoea often have been infected with *Chlamydia* at the same time, it is usual to follow the penicillin tablets with a ten-day course of tablets of an antibiotic called doxycycline or two days of a newer antibiotic called azithromycin.

One month after treatment the woman must return for a further check (when swabs are taken from her cervix and from her urethra) to make sure that she is cured.

Syphilis

Syphilis is the least common but potentially the most serious of the sexually transmitted diseases. Unless it is cured, it could lead to a painful death or mental decay ten to twenty years later. Syphilis is caused by a tiny cork-screw shaped germ, called the *Treponema pallidum* (TP). TP enters the skin of the labia during sexual intercourse with a man who has a syphilitic ulcer on his penis. After an interval of three to seven weeks, it causes an ulcer on the woman's vulva or her cervix. The discharge from the ulcer teems with TP and is very infectious.

If the woman visits a doctor, a swab will be taken from the ulcer and the pathologist will be able to see the TP through a microscope. Syphilis is cured by injections of penicillin. After treatment the woman has to return for further tests at intervals. At each visit a blood test is taken. If the tests are negative after a year, the woman is cured. If the tests are positive, further courses of treatment are given.

AIDS

AIDS is short for acquired immune deficiency syndrome. AIDS is caused by a virus, the human immunodeficiency virus (HIV). HIV infection is becoming increasingly common all over the world. In Africa and Asia most cases occur when a man is infected after having sex with a prostitute, and then infects his wife or other sexual partners. In Western countries most cases were originally reported among homosexual men and intra-venous drug-users, but recently increasing numbers of cases are occurring among sexually active heterosexual men and women.

The HIV enters the body during sexual intercourse through tiny cracks in the lining of the vagina, the penis, or the rectum (if you have anal intercourse) or is transferred in infected blood if drug-users share needles. It can also be transferred by blood transfusion of infected blood.

In the body the virus causes a minor, flu-like episode and then remains quiet, causing no symptoms for up to ten years. During this time, however, the person can infect others with whom he or she has sexual intercourse. Some years after the initial infection the virus becomes active and damages the white blood cells, which help to protect the body against infection. In consequence a variety of infections occur, and sometimes cancer occurs; pro-gressively, the person becomes increasingly ill and dies.

The disease can be detected by a blood test within three months of the original infection. The blood test shows that the person has been infected but tells nothing about how long the

---

Facts about HIV infection and AIDS

There are a lot of myths about HIV infection, but the following information should destroy many of these harmful beliefs.

- You can't get AIDS by casual contact with a person who has AIDS.
- You will not get AIDS if you shake hands, hug, or kiss a person who has AIDS.
- You will not get AIDS if you use a toilet or a telephone that an AIDS patient has used.
- You will not get AIDS if you share crockery, cutlery, towels, sheets, or linen with a person who has AIDS.
- You can't catch AIDS by talking to, or cuddling, a person who is AIDS antibody positive, as the virus will only infect you if you have anal intercourse, very active vaginal intercourse, or perhaps oral sex with an infected person, when bodily fluids are exchanged.

infection will remain dormant or how soon the symptoms of AIDS will occur. Currently, it is believed that more than 60 per cent of HIV-infected people will develop symptoms and will become seriously ill within ten years of contracting HIV.

When symptoms occur, AIDS goes through two stages. In the first stage—the 'AIDS–related complex'—the person's glands swell, and he or she has night sweats, always feels tired, and loses weight. After a number of months the symptoms clear up, but one person in three will develop the severe, terminal stage of AIDS in the next one to three years. In the severe stage of AIDS, the person is extremely ill, and more than three-quarters of those in this stage will die within a year.

There is no cure for AIDS at present, although there are several drugs that will delay the progress of the disease.

Avoiding HIV infection

You can avoid getting infected by HIV and developing AIDS if you avoid having sexual intercourse or sharing needles. Only a few people use intravenous drugs, but many young people (and older people) have had sex with more than one partner. A study in the UK reported in 1991 that one in four people aged 18–20 had had at least one new sexual partner in the previous year and did not take precautions against HIV infection.

The first precaution is to insist that the man uses a condom when you have sex, unless you are absolutely sure that he has not had sex with other men or women before meeting you, or that he has had a blood test that was negative for HIV/AIDS. (That applies to you, too: if you have had sex with other men you should make sure that your new partner uses a condom for his protection, or you should have an HIV blood test.) If you follow these suggestions you are practising 'safer sex' and have little or no risk of developing HIV infection.

Unfortunately, the British survey showed that only 5 per cent of the young people insisted that their male sexual partner wore a condom each time they had sex, and a third of the people surveyed believed that only drug-users and homosexual men were at risk of being infected with HIV. The good news is that things are improving. Today in the UK, more young people are using condoms than any other kind of contraceptive. Two-thirds of the men surveyed said that women should carry condoms, and only 2 per cent of the men reported that they were embarrassed by buying condoms. HIV infection and AIDS will only be controlled if sexually active people practise 'safer sex'.

Control of sexually transmitted diseases

Obviously if no person ever had sex with another person except his or her permanent partner, then sexually transmitted diseases would cease to be a problem. However, at no time in history has this occurred.

If you really want to have sexual intercourse, you can reduce your chances of catching an STD if you follow these guidelines:

- Limit the number of partners that you have.
- Talk with your partner before you have sex to find out if there is any chance of him having an STD. If he has, and wants sex with you and will not wear a condom, he doesn't love you—he is exploiting you.
- If you have several partners, go and see a doctor every six months and have a check to make sure you don't have an STD.
- Try to talk your partner into having checks to make sure he (or they) does not have an STD.
- If you have sex with a partner you don't know very well, try to make sure he uses a condom as this reduces the chance that he will infect you with gonorrhoea, *Chlamydia*, or HIV infection.

Chapter Thirteen

Looking good, feeling good

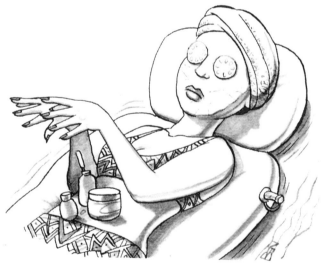

Everything has its beauty but not everyone sees it.

Confucius

Most teenagers want to feel good and to look good. When you feel good, you generally look good. Your personality shines out, and other people see you as being a real person. You relate better to other people, and they want to relate to you. When you feel good, you become more outgoing and interested in what goes on around you. You smile more, you are more animated. You feel that life is interesting and worth living.

- People feel good if they eat a nutritious diet, as discussed in chapter 6.
- People feel good if they can cope with any psychological upsets that they might have (see chapter 15).
- People feel good if they take regular exercise that they enjoy.
- People feel good if they and others think they look good.

These last two matters are discussed in this chapter.

Exercise

Most people, including teenagers, do not take much exercise unless they are forced to do so or are convinced that exercise will benefit their health. A recent study in Australia asked a thousand randomly selected men and women about the amount of physical activity they undertook. The researchers also asked the people whether they thought that their health would be improved if they exercised regularly. A quarter of the people interviewed said that they would feel healthier if they exercised more. They were then asked why they were not exercising more. Half the people responded by saying that they had no time, and a third that they were too lazy.

Regular exercise improves the function of your heart. It also keeps muscles strong and joints flexible and, if incorporated into a weight reduction program, enables an overweight person to lose weight more quickly. In fact, regular exercise usually makes a person feel good. A reason for this is that exercise increases the release of endorphins (opium-like substances) from your brain, which gives you a 'high'.

There are two main kinds of exercise. The first is designed to improve the performance of your heart and lungs. This is achieved by aerobic exercises. The second kind of exercises are designed to strengthen your muscles and are adopted by body-builders. These exercises might give you strong pectoral muscles if you pump iron, and in consequence might make your breasts more prominent, but they are less beneficial to your health than are aerobic exercises.

If you are still at school it is likely that you will be doing physical education classes and playing some sport. These programs all keep you fit. But if you do additional exercises you will be even fitter.

There are several principles of an exercise program:

- You should choose an exercise or sport that you enjoy.
- The exercises should be graded and increased gradually.
- The exercises should not produce severe discomfort. The idea of 'no pain, no gain' is ridiculous. Your body knows best.
- In most cases you should start with a warm-up period and end with a cool-down period. During your warm up and cool down you should stretch muscle groups gently to reduce the chance of injuring them.

Looking good

When a person looks at you they look first at your face and then at your body. If your face is animated and your skin is clear, people will respond to your appealing appearance. Most teenagers are worried about how their skin looks and whether they have acne. Acne is discussed specifically in chapter 14; this chapter discusses general skin and health care.

Skin

'There is no magician's mantle to compare with the skin in its diverse roles of waterproof, overcoat, sunshade, suit of armour and refrigerator, sensitive to the touch of a feather, to temperature and pain, withstanding the wear and tear of three score years and ten, and executing its own running repairs.' Thus wrote the anatomist R.D. Lockhart in 1956, in a description of the skin that could hardly be bettered.

The skin varies in thickness. On the eyelids it is only 0.5 mm thick, but on the soles of the feet it is 4 mm thick or more. In places such as the palms of the hands and on the ears, the skin is firmly bound to the underlying structures. But the skin covering most of the body is freely movable. It is smooth or rough, dry or moist, depending on the number of sweat and sebaceous glands it contains. Most of it is covered with hair, which could be soft and downy, scarcely perceptible, or it could be coarse and long. In youth, the skin is firm and elastic; in old age, it is often loose and wrinkled. It holds a mirror to your health, changing in its appearance when you are ill. This vital organ, roughly 1.7 square metres in extent, covers your body, protecting and isolating it from the environment.

The skin consists of two layers, the epidermis and the dermis, and both are of equal importance (see figure 13.1). The epidermis, the layer in contact with the environment, is made up of layers of cells, all of which are derived from the deeper layer, the dermis. As the cells mature, they change in shape and in character and are pushed towards the surface of your body, when they lose their boundaries and their nuclei and become a thickened, callous layer. In this layer, which varies in thickness, dead cells· are constantly being shed from the surface—more than 9 grams are lost each day, mostly invisibly, but sometimes embarrassingly as dandruff. This callous, horny layer is vital for life because it is the waterproof layer of your skin. However, certain medications, hormones, and poisons can enter the body through the skin, so its waterproofing capability is not perfect.

The pigmentation of the skin is due to tiny particles of a substance called melanin in the deepest layers of the epidermis. The more melanin, the darker the skin. Melanin protects the skin against the damaging effects of sunlight, which is why 'white'-skinned people tan when exposed to sunlight. Unfortunately, the skin itself can be damaged by this exposure, although the tissues beneath it are protected.

The dermis is a felted meshwork of fibrous and elastic tissues, and it is riveted to the epidermis by projections that stud its surface. In it blood, lymph vessels, and nerves find their way. The fibrous tissue is mainly formed from a protein called collagen. In the dermis are found the roots of the hairs, with their accompanying sebaceous glands and the sweat glands, all of which open on the skin's surface through narrow tubes.

The skin is a restless organ, constantly rearranging itself, constantly shedding surface cells and making new cells. Through it hairs, themselves made up of dead cells, grow, increase in length, live for about two years, and are replaced by new hairs growing from the hair follicle deep in the dermis. The

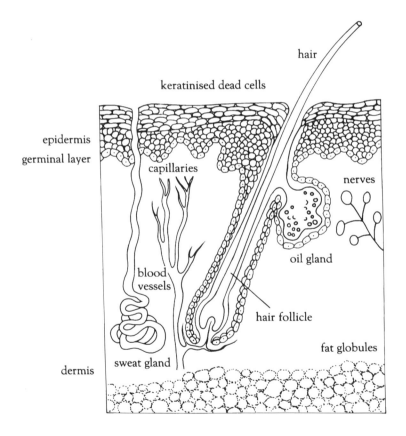

Figure 13.1 The structure of the skin.

sebaceous glands are constantly active, secreting the oil-like sebum, which is similar to the lanolin of sheep's wool and which greases the surface of the body, keeping the skin pliable. If a gland-making sebum becomes blocked, a whitehead, a blackhead or a small cyst will result (see chapter 14).

Hair follicles

The hair follicles are narrow tubes, each of which contains a single hair. Only the root of the hair is alive: the rest is made up of dead, keratinised (horny) cells. The hair grows as its root creates new cells, which push the cells overlying them upwards towards the surface of the skin. As the cells are pushed upwards, they become keratinised. A small muscle is attached to each hair follicle. When this muscle contracts, the hair becomes erect, and the skin above the muscle bunches up to make a 'goose bump'. These changes occur if a person is cold or suddenly frightened. Each hair follicle has a sebaceous or oil gland attached to it. The oil is secreted into the tube of the hair follicle and lubricates it. It also washes out the cells that line the follicle when they die. The oil seeps out of each hair follicle and covers the skin surface with a very thin layer of oil, called sebum. As oil is removed by constant rubbing of the skin from movement or clothes, or is evaporated by sunlight, more sebum emerges from the sebaceous glands to replace it. Hair follicles are found in all parts of the skin except on the palms of the hands, the soles of the feet, the lips, and the eyelids.

The amount of hair on your body, its fineness or coarseness, depends on your racial group and on the genes you have inherited. Some races, such as the Chinese, produce only fine, scanty body hair. Other races, such as Mediterranean people, tend to have a lot of coarse body hair. A few women develop coarse hair on parts of the body where it is usually found only in men. These women might grow a moustache or even a beard. This kind of hair grows because the women are especially sensitive to, or have produced abnormal quantities of, the male sex hormone testosterone. A few women grow hair on their breasts in the area of the nipple. These are of no consequence but might cause concern. If they do, you can pluck them.

Sweat glands

Sweat glands are found in the dermis of the skin and reach the skin's surface through a narrow tube. There are two kinds of sweat glands in your skin. The first, which are called eccrine sweat glands, are found in most parts of the skin, but are found in greater numbers on the forehead, the palms, and the armpits. The eccrine glands secrete salt and water, which is why sweat tastes salty. The eccrine glands help to regulate the temperature of your body. When your body gets hot, either because it is a hot, humid day, or because of exercise, you sweat. The sweat is released from the eccrine glands into the skin's surface and cools it by evaporation. Anxiety, excitement, or fear can also lead to sweating; people 'break out in a cold sweat'. This means that, because of nervous stress, their eccrine glands start to secrete sweat.

The second kind of sweat glands have a different structure and function, and are called apocrine sweat glands. These glands are only found in the armpits and the genital area. They appear only after puberty and produce sweat, which, on exposure to air, has a musky smell. In less advanced mammals, the smell is a sexual attraction, but humans have lost the sensitive sense of smell and only notice it when they are very close to a sexually aroused person.

Nerves

If you touch an object you can tell whether it is rough or smooth, hot or cold, painful or pleasant. These sensations are possible because the dermis has many nerve fibres that relay these sensations from your skin to your brain. Different nerve fibres carry different messages to the brain. The nerve fibres also surround the hair follicles, which is why it hurts when you pull out a hair.

Blood vessels

With this degree of complexity, the skin needs a good blood supply to carry oxygen and energy to it and remove waste products from it. The blood vessels in the skin form a network of fine, thin-walled vessels called capillaries. Capillaries have muscles in their walls, which can contract to shut the capillary down so that heat is not lost from your body in cold weather. In hot weather, when your body temperature rises, the capillaries dilate. An increased amount of blood flows through them, and this enables heat to be lost through the epidermis. If you are embarrassed, the capillaries dilate and you blush.

Skin care

The skin is such a complex organ that it needs to be looked after carefully to keep it in good condition. The superficial layers of cells are shed constantly; bacteria live on the skin's surface in their millions; the oil secreted by the hair follicles mixes with the shed, dead skin cells and dust. Unless you get rid of this mess, your skin will look dirty and you will feel uncomfortable.

The best way of cleansing the skin is to use soap. Soap breaks down the oil into tiny droplets, which then release the matted, dead skin cells and allow the skin's surface to become clean. If you prefer, you can pay a bit more and use a cleansing skin cream or lotion. Skin creams and lotions are not skin foods, whatever the manufacturers say, as they are not absorbed through the skin. They break down the oily mass on the skin so that it can be washed or wiped away.

Moisturisers

Some creams and lotions are made to keep the skin moist rather than to clean it. In normal conditions the oil secreted by the sebaceous glands keeps the skin surface moist by holding water in its meshwork as a sort of glue. But in windy, dry weather, or as you grow older, the moisture is lost and the skin might become rough and dry. If this happens, a moisturising cream can be applied to areas of skin that are exposed to the weather. These are usually the face and the back of the hands. If you have dry skin, apply a moisturiser when you have washed your hands and let the moisturised area dry in the air.

Manufacturers of cosmetics offer a large and bewildering range of lotions and creams that moisten the skin, reduce the dry feeling, and perhaps delay the formation of wrinkles. The cost of moisturisers varies enormously, as does their effectiveness. In the opinion of the user, effectiveness ranges from 'well above average' to 'well below average', according to a survey of seventy-two products conducted by the Australian Consumers' Association. The conclusion of the survey was that moisturisers do help dry skin, but that the effectiveness of the moisturiser bears no relation to its cost: a cheap moisturiser headed the list. Nor was there any relationship between the effectiveness of the product, the user's age, the climatic conditions, or the user's skin type. This means that, according to the ACA, you waste money if you buy a moisturiser that is especially expensive, or said to be ideal for young skin, or for special weathers and seasons, or especially for 'combination' skin. Nor are night creams any more effective than other moisturisers.

Large numbers of women, persuaded by skilled advertising, purchase creams, lotions, skin tonics, and hormone preparation to delay wrinkles and other signs of the ageing process in the skin. The products are lavishly launched, superbly packaged, seductively perfumed, and often very expensive. Do they do what they claim to do, namely delay the inevitable changes that occur in the skin as a woman ages? The answer is that they do not. The best way to keep the skin in good condition is by cleaning it regularly, using soap and water, and drying it carefully. There is no cosmetic that will keep your skin youthful if your genetic inheritance decrees that it will age quickly. You might abuse your skin in youth by excessive sunbathing, which will hurry the process of ageing (and might also cause skin cancer), but it is unlikely that the moisturising creams produced to limit the effects of that abuse are of any more benefit than the use of a cheap vaseline or lanolin product, which will help the skin look smooth and soft, and is just as effective as a more expensive moisturiser.

If buying expensive skin products makes you feel good, by all means buy them. The product will do no harm except to your pocket, and will probably do as much good as a cheaper product you can buy from any chemist.

Getting a tan

Until recently, most young women (and many older women) believed that if you had a good tan you were more attractive. Lying in the sun, particularly at the beach, made you relaxed and warm and at the same time gave you a wonderful tan.

It now appears that by lying in the sun we could be doing ourselves a good deal of harm. Not only are we increasing our chance of developing facial wrinkles in middle age, but we are also increasing our chance of developing skin cancer.

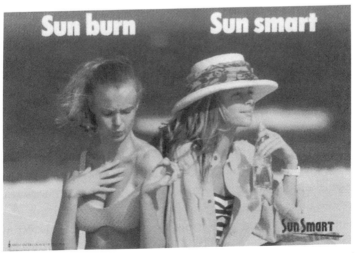

Despite the facts and the advertising, many people still get sunburnt as they pursue a 'healthy' tan and the risk of skin cancer is increased.

This knowledge has led to a new concept: keep out of the sun if you can. If you go out in the sun for any time longer than 15 minutes, *slip* on a shirt, *slap* on a hat with a wide brim, *slop* on a layer of protective sun screen, and wrap on sunglasses.

Sunlight is made up of visible light—the light that looks white but in reality is all the colours that make up a rainbow. The colours are red, orange, yellow, green, blue, indigo, and violet. Beyond the red end of the spectrum there is infra-red light, which we feel as heat. Beyond the violet end of the spectrum is a light we can't see but which has high energy and can penetrate the skin. This is ultraviolet (UV) light. Ultraviolet light, better called ultraviolet radiation, penetrates the skin to varying depths and causes chemical reactions. For example, if you look directly at the sun for even one second, the ultraviolet rays might so damage the cells at the back of your eye that you become blind. The amount of penetration of your skin by ultraviolet rays depends on the number of melanocytes that you have in your epidermis. Dark-skinned people have many melanocytes; fair-skinned people have few melanocytes. Melanocytes produce skin pigment granules called melanin, which absorb the ultraviolet rays and prevent them from damaging other parts of the skin, especially the dermis.

What happens when you lie in the sun?

First, the ultraviolet rays affect your epidermis. If you have a lot of pigment cells, most of the energy from the ultraviolet light is absorbed by them; if you are fair-skinned, most of the ultraviolet light penetrates through the epidermis to reach the dermis. The ultraviolet light also stimulates the growth of new cells, so that the epidermis is thickened. If the exposure to the sun is sudden, the epidermis might thicken quickly and the superficial layer might crack and peel off. If the exposure to the sun occurs often, the thickened epidermis does not peel, and the skin becomes leathery and wrinkled.

Some of the ultraviolet radiation penetrates the epidermis and reaches the dermis. Small amounts of sunlight are beneficial, as the rays produce vitamin D from chemicals found in the cells of the dermis. But if you lie in the sun and become sunburnt, the ultraviolet radiation can damage the cells. The radiation produces energy and heats the tissues. The body reacts to this and tries to get rid of the heat by increasing the blood supply and dilating the capillaries. Fluid also seeps into the tissues of the dermis. At first, as you lie in the sun, you feel a warm 'glow'. It feels good. If you lie too long, the glow is replaced by a reddened, tender, swollen skin. You are sunburnt.

Repeated exposure to the sun in this way leads to damage of the elastic fibres and the collagen in the dermis. These fibres become damaged, and the skin becomes prematurely wrinkled.

It is useful to remember that ultraviolet radiation is not felt as heat: it is 'cold'. You can become sunburnt when there is no heat in the sun, and on overcast days, as the ultraviolet rays penetrate light cloud. You can also get sunburnt if you avoid the direct sun but forget that the sunlight is reflected by the sea, the sand, and the snow. You can also damage your skin when you use a solarium to tan your body as a solarium produces ultraviolet rays.

Limiting damage caused by sunlight

If you live in a hot, sunny country it is best to acquire the habit of using a sunscreen or moisturiser containing a sunscreen on your face and hands every day.

Even though the experts tell us that we should avoid exposure to the sun, many young women still continue to lie in the sun for long periods of time. How can the damage be reduced?

First, avoid lying in the sun when its rays are strongest, that is, between the hours of 11 a.m. and 3 p.m. Second, if you must sunbake, expose your body to the sun for a short period of time at first, and increase the exposure gradually. How long your first exposure should be depends on your skin, and the number and activity of the melanocytes in the dermis. Third, make sure that the exposed parts of your body are covered with a protective sunscreen, which has a sun protection factor (SPF) of at least 15.

The SPF is found by: the time to achieve minimal noticeable redness with the cream applied *divided* by the time to produce the same amount of redness with no cream. The higher the SPF, the more protective is the sunscreen. A lotion or a cream with an SPF of 10 means that on average a person can be in the sun for ten times longer than if she used no sunscreen. This is a bit misleading as a sunscreen that should prevent sunburn for ten hours on an average day when it is applied to the skin at 9 a.m. does not offer the same protection at 3 p.m. And remember that some ultraviolet radiation will always be transmitted even through sunscreens with the highest SPF.

The protection afforded by a sunscreen does not only depend on its SPF, it also depends on how evenly you apply the sunscreen, how thickly you apply it, and how often. One application will not protect you for the entire day. The sunscreen absorbs ultraviolet radiation and is changed chemically. The sunscreen is washed off when you sweat or swim. In fact, a wet skin, whether from sweat, a shower, or a swim, enables ultraviolet radiation to penetrate the skin more deeply.

But neither keeping out of the sun between 11 a.m. and 3 p.m., nor using protective waterproof sunscreens is as protective as the 'Slip, Slop, Slap, Wrap' policy recommended by anti-cancer councils.

Hair

The romantic poets wrote, 'Hair is a woman's crowning glory'. So it is if it is clean and shining; it is not if it is dirty. Most women take care of their hair, but problems can arise.

Dull and greasy hair

Every day scales of skin are shed beneath your hair. Every day greasy oil is secreted by the hair follicles. On your scalp the greasy oil matts with the scales of skin and with dust from the atmosphere. The mixture fixes to your hair, which becomes greasy, loses its glistening look, and might become itchy. Your hair needs washing.

You can wash your hair with soap, or you might prefer to use a shampoo. Shampoos come with a bewildering range of additives and prices. Most rely on a substance that breaks down the oily greasy substances attached to the hairs into tiny droplets, which can then be washed away by rinsing. Rinsing is important. Without it, the droplets would remain and recombine to form greasy oil. Shampoos also have a foaming action that enables the active substance to reach all the greasy areas. At the end of a shampoo the hair is clean but has no natural oils as they have been rinsed away. Because of this, many people use a hair 'conditioner' after shampooing. The conditioner makes the hair less tangled and enables it to settle down better after a shampoo.

Dandruff

If your scalp is dry, the shed scales of skin might not be caught in your scalp oil. If this happens, from time to time you will shed showers of scales, called dandruff. If regular hair care does not control the dandruff, you could try one of the anti-dandruff formulae. (Ask your pharmacist.)

Chapter
Fourteen

Teenage medical problems

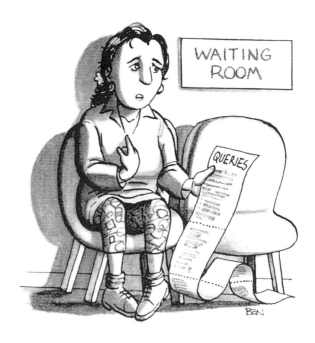

Zits are the pits!

Slogan

Like any other group in the population, teenage women visit their doctor when they feel ill. Many of these visits are for coughs, colds, and other illnesses, but teenage women have some special reasons for visiting a doctor. In studies conducted in Sydney and Boston, the following were most often quoted by adolescent women as areas in which they needed help:

- contraceptive advice
- menstrual cramps
- weight and eating problems
- acne
- vaginal discharges
- menstrual disturbances
- hyperventilation
- exercise and exercise disorders.

The first three medical problems are discussed elsewhere in this book (see chapters 9, 4, and 7, respectively); the others are considered here.

Acne

At puberty there is an increase in the activity of the grease-producing (sebaceous) glands of the skin. The increased activity is probably due to the effects of the sex hormones (particularly the male sex hormone, testosterone), which are now being produced in the body. As well as producing more grease (sebum) in the gland itself, for some reason the cells lining the duct that connects the gland to the surface of the skin start multiplying, with the result that the duct narrows and might become blocked. If this occurs, a whitehead is formed (see figure 14.1). If the duct remains open, although narrowed, the gland continues to expand as more sebum is produced, and the duct fills with sebum which dries, forming a keratin plug. When the keratin plug meets the air, it turns black. The result is a blackhead, which, although unsightly, can be controlled by gentle removal.

Whiteheads are the cause of many of the problems and much of the unsightliness of acne. The gland continues to produce sebum, which cannot escape because the duct is blocked. Inside the gland, bacteria called *Propionibacterium* acne (or the acne organism) act on the sebum, converting some of it to irritating fatty acids. Eventually the gland bursts, expelling the fatty acids (and bacteria) into the surrounding tissue. This results in a pustule or, if deeper in the skin, in a tender, inflamed pimple. Some of these pustules and swellings are converted into scar tissue during the healing process, leaving the pits sometimes seen on the face or neck of an acne sufferer.

Acne occurs most commonly on the face, neck, chest, shoulders, and back, and it can be aggravated by emotional stress. Lying in the sun to get a good tan might aggravate acne because the skin reacts to mild sunburn by adding skin cells in its surface, and these cells might block sebaceous glands. Treating acne by rubbing the skin hard has the same effect. If you have acne, don't do either. Its presence can, in turn, cause great emotional distress, particularly as the condition is more common during adolescence. Between 60 and 80 per cent of teenagers are affected, 15 per cent severely. Acne usually ceases by the age of 25, but some people continue to develop new lesions of acne into their thirties or forties.

Acne is not caused by eating rich or fatty foods, and dietary restrictions, such as cutting out sugar and fats, have proved ineffective. Acne is not due to poor personal hygiene, to lack of

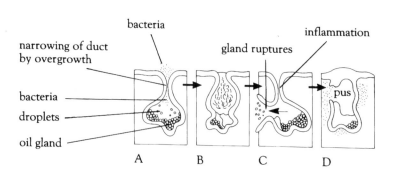

Figure 14.1 The formation of a pimple. (a) Duct narrows, bacteria multiply. (b) Inflamed pimple. (c) Whitehead (blocked duct). (d) Pustule.

exercise, to overindulgence in alcohol, or to masturbation. It is not caused by an oily skin; in fact an oily skin is an advantage.

Until recently, the treatment for acne has been relatively unsatisfactory, and even today there is no specific treatment. The principles of treatment are: first, to reduce the numbers of bacteria (and fatty acids) in the skin glands; second, to contain the excessive growth of the cells lining the ducts; and finally, to eliminate the whiteheads, pustules, and nodules.

Acne can be controlled, to some extent, if the person uses a pH neutral cleanser to wash the affected area. This does not aggravate the skin and they are available in supermarkets and pharmacies. Your pharmacist or doctor can help you if you feel unsure about what may help. Scrubbing the affected skin is not advised. If acne affects the face, thick make-up should be avoided and a non-medicated lightweight, non-greasy make-up chosen. If the acne is bad, the psychological benefit of using make-up could be considerable.

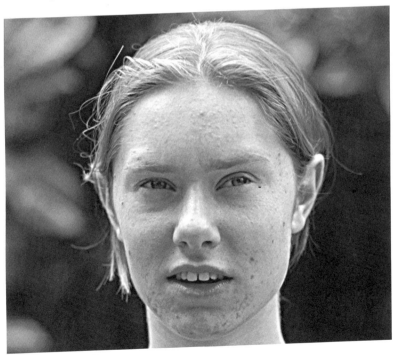

A severe case of acne.

Mild acne generally only needs to be treated with medications applied to the affected areas of the skin. If mild acne doesn't respond to the pH neutral cleanser, then an oral contraceptive (the pill) often helps. For moderately severe acne, a treatment consisting of a drug that counteracts the effects of testosterone (called cyproterone) and an oestrogen is available. The drug, taken for twenty-one days each month, has reduced the number of acne lumps by half after four months' treatment. The drug seems to be more effective than the pill. Another treatment is to take a drug called spironalactone, or to rub an ointment containing it on the parts of the skin affected by acne. The drug has to be used daily for three to six months to be effective.

If a teenager has acne with many pustules, other treatments can be tried. One of the most helpful is a combined treatment of antibiotics and application of a lotion to the affected area. The antibiotics chosen are tetracycline or erythromycin. Both are relatively cheap and free from side-effects. As it takes up to three weeks for the antibiotic to penetrate the glands, the drugs have to be given for a minimum of four weeks and are usually continued for six months. At the same time the teenager applies a lotion or gel of 5 per cent benzyl peroxide to the acne area. Benzyl peroxide inhibits the growth of the acne organism and reduces the production of the fatty acids in the gland. The drug has to be prescribed by a doctor, and its use is medically supervised as it might be irritating to the skin.

If the acne is very severe, particularly if it is lumpy (cystic), if scarring is occurring, if it is disfiguring, extensive, or painful, another drug, called isotretinoin, might be suggested by the doctor. The drug is derived from retinoic acid (vitamin A). Isotretinoin (Roacutain) makes the cells lining the duct less 'sticky' so that they are expelled from the duct more easily. This permits the blocked duct to reopen. The drug also reduces the production of sebum.

Isotretinoin is a potentially dangerous drug and must be given under careful medical supervision, as it can cause dry lips, a dry mouth, or eye irritation. It should never be given to a woman who is pregnant as it could cause congenital defects in the baby. Tablets of isotretinoin are taken by mouth twice per day for three months if the severe acne disfigures the face, and for four months if the severe cystic acne affects the body (usually the back and the chest).

Vaginal discharges

The vagina starts at the hymen and extends upwards and backwards to reach the uterus. It is a muscular 'tube', although in reality its walls lie close to each other unless the vagina is distended by a finger, a tampon, a man's penis or a baby being born. In other words, the vagina can stretch considerably when necessary.

The vagina is a remarkable organ. Not only is it capable of great distension but it also keeps itself clean. The walls of the vagina are formed by cells that lie on top of each other in a layer twenty cells deep, like the bricks of a house wall. During the reproductive years, when oestrogen is circulating in large quantities in a woman's body, the top cells are constantly shed into the vagina. There, a small bacillus acts on the separated cells to produce lactic acid. The lactic acid kills most contaminating germs that happen to get into the vagina.

During the reproductive years the vagina is kept moist by fluid that seeps between the cells making up its walls. This keeps the vagina healthy and flexible. If a woman is aroused sexually, the amount of fluid is increased and the vagina becomes wet. In older women, who do not secrete oestrogen, the fluid is not formed and the vagina becomes dry and uncomfortable.

The fluid, the exfoliated vaginal cells (called 'exfoliated' because they are shed like leaves from a tree), and the lactic acid combine to produce a small amount of whitish secretion, which has a 'fishy' odour. If the woman is under stress, or anxious or for other reasons, the amount of the 'whites' (the medical name is leukorrhoea) might increase, might become clotted, and can cause discomfort or an itch.

If the vaginal discharge is sufficient to make a young woman anxious she should visit a doctor. This is especially so if the vagina becomes itchy or the discharge is very smelly, as it might be due to a vaginal infection. Infective discharges are of three kinds:

- those caused by a fungus called *Candida*, or thrush
- those caused by a tiny single-celled animal called trichomonad
- those caused by a bacterium called *Gardnerella* interacting with anaerobic (not needing oxygen) germs. This infection is called bacterial vaginosis or non-specific vaginitis.

The only way a doctor can tell which of these infections has occurred is to take a swab from the vagina. The doctor does this by looking into the vagina with a speculum and gently scraping the vaginal wall with a cotton-wool bud on a stick. The discharge collected is then placed in a container and sent to a pathology laboratory for analysis.

Candida

Candida infections of the vagina, which are also known as monilia and thrush, are caused by a fungus. *Candida* is found in the vagina of between 5 and 25 per cent of women aged between 15 and 50. In most women *Candida* does not cause any symptoms as its growth is kept in check by the other bacteria that live in the vagina. But occasionally, if a change in the vaginal environment occurs, perhaps because of stress, because the woman has been taking antibiotics, or has had sexual intercourse with a man who has *Candida* infection of his penis, the fungus starts growing. When this happens an irritating vaginal discharge will appear. Between 2 and 4 per cent of young women develop the infection. The discharge is usually whitish in colour, and the itch might involve the woman's vagina and her vulva. *Candida* is diagnosed by taking a swab from the vagina, and sending it to a pathology laboratory where it is inoculated into a culture medium in which the fungus grows quickly.

Treatment is easy. The woman puts cream or a tablet of an anti-fungal drug in her vagina either for three or for six days. This cures more than 85 per cent of women. If the infection recurs, the doctor might repeat the treatment or give tablets to be taken by mouth. The reason is that in some cases the thrush lives in the woman's bowel and is transferred from the anus to the vagina. After opening her bowels a woman should always wipe herself from front to back to avoid the possible transfer of *Candida*.

Trichomoniasis

Trichomoniasis is due to a single-celled animal, the trichomonad. It is the size of a pus cell, and it infects the vagina of between 2 and 20 per cent of women aged between 15 and 50. In most cases the animals are transmitted sexually. In a man, trichomoniasis usually does not cause any symptoms, but it can cause an itchy vaginal discharge in women when there is a change in the vaginal environment. If a swab is taken from the woman's vagina, the trichomonads can be seen through a microscope. If the doctor is in any doubt, the swab is sent to a laboratory and smeared on a culture medium.

Treatment of trichomoniasis is to take a single dose of four tablets of a special drug (called Fasigyn) or one tablet of metronidazole (Flagyl) three times per day for seven days.

Non-specific vaginitis

Also called bacterial vaginosis or anaerobic vaginosis, non-specific vaginitis is a vaginal discharge that is greyish in colour and smells strongly 'fishy'. The discharge is due to the interaction of bacteria that normally live in the vagina. The diagnosis is made when the doctor takes a swab from the vagina and sends it to a pathology laboratory for analysis. The treatment of non-specific vaginal discharge is the same as the treatment for trichomoniasis or an antibacterial cream (Dalacin V) can be used. Some creams help to restore the acidity of the vagina and these may help. Douching or inserting yoghurt is not advised; these reduce the natural defences of the vagina to 'help itself'

Menstrual disturbances

Between 5 and 10 per cent of teenage women visit a doctor because of menstrual disturbances. A woman might worry that her menstrual periods are occurring too often or too infrequently. They might seem to her to be too heavy or too light. In most cases the disturbance to the menstrual cycle is that the periods are unpredictable. In a few cases the periods are irregular at the time of onset but, when they come, are heavy and prolonged.

It is useful for a teenage woman to note in her diary when her menstrual periods start and when they stop, so that she has a 'menstrual calendar'. If the disturbance is minor, the doctor generally will give reassurance rather than drugs. If the disturbance is severe, the doctor will make blood tests and usually prescribe the oral contraceptive pill to regulate the menstrual cycle and reduce the menstrual blood loss. In most cases this is enough to regulate the periods. A few young women (about one in twenty of those who have had a severe menstrual disturbance) will continue to have episodes of heavy, irregular bleeding, and will need to be investigated further.

Hyperventilation

Hyperventilation is the medical term for overbreathing, usually by taking rapid shallow breaths. The effect of overbreathing is to reduce the level of carbon dioxide gas in your blood and, often, to lower the level of blood calcium. These changes in your metabolism cause symptoms. You might develop numbness around your mouth, tingling in your fingers or toes, or dizziness. In severe overbreathing you might develop cramps in your hands. Overbreathing also causes mental disturbances. You might develop a feeling of extreme anxiety or unreality as your consciousness clouds. And this could make you hyperventilate more. Chronic hyperventilators often feel fatigued easily and might faint.

Hyperventilation can be very frightening. You can overcome it, however. If you develop the symptoms of finger tingling or mouth numbness, or feelings of anxiety and fright, sit down and relax. Then slow down your breathing; take a normal but slow breath in counting to four, hold this breath counting slowly to four, release this breath and breathe out counting to four. Next try counting to five or six. If you can't relax, get a small paper bag, put it over your mouth and nose, and breathe in and out. You will find that the strange symptoms disappear quite quickly. And then you will be able to slow down your breathing. By slowing the rate at which you breathe, or by breathing into the paper bag, you increase the level of carbon dioxide in your blood, and so relieve the symptoms of hyperventilation.

Exercise and exercise disorders

A teenage woman's health benefits if she takes exercise regularly, participating in some sort of sport—dancing, gymnastics, cycling, running, etc. If she is at school she will probably have an exercise program she has to follow, but when she leaves school she has to decide for herself whether she will continue to exercise. She might continue to exercise to keep fit, because she enjoys the sport, or because she wants to be slim and to change her body appearance.

The desire to be slim and fit has led some women to become so preoccupied with exercise and body shape that they spend many hours each day exercising. If they exercise excessively before puberty they might delay the onset of menstruation by two or more years. Teenage women who have started menstruating sometimes find that their periods cease when they exercise excessively, particularly if they also restrict the amount of food they eat. This could have negative consequences for the woman's health. The exercise and food restriction stop the hypothalamus sending hormonal messages to the pituitary gland (see the section on puberty in chapter 3). This prevents the pituitary gland from making and releasing the follicle-stimulating hormone into the blood. Deprived of this hormone, the ovaries stop producing oestrogen, and menstruation ceases. If the oestrogen deprivation continues for six months or longer, it not only prevents menstruation but also stops the bones from increasing their density and becoming stronger, at a time when the bone mass is increasing most rapidly. As a result, the peak bone mass, which is normally reached when a woman is 30, might be less than it normally would be, and this can increase the chance that the woman will develop osteoporosis in middle age. (Regular, *moderate* exercise throughout a woman's life, however, increases bone density and reduces the likelihood of the onset of osteoporosis.)

To prevent the possibility of this harmful effect on bone density and strength, a teenager who exercises excessively, and is younger than 16 and not menstruating, should reduce the amount of exercise she takes and ensure that she eats a nutritious diet. She should then begin to menstruate. A woman older than 16 should take the same action as well as consider going on the pill, which will provide the oestrogen her ovaries are not making.

A few teenage women develop a disorder in which exercise becomes the all-consuming passion of their life. They are so obsessed by exercise that they might give up promising careers and courses of study to work out in gyms or sporting venues. They say that they cannot stop exercising because exercise makes them feel good and puts them 'on a high'. But to keep 'on a high' they have to keep increasing the amount of exercise they do. Some of these women feel compelled to exercise even if they are ill or injured. They continue their exercise program every day, even if they have to go without sleep.

A few women who have an exercise disorder have a coexisting eating disorder. Some women alternate between episodes of disordered eating and disordered exercise.

If you feel that you might have or could be developing an exercise disorder, you should consult your doctor, who will be able to help you establish a moderate, healthy exercise program.

Chapter Fifteen

Teenage psychological problems

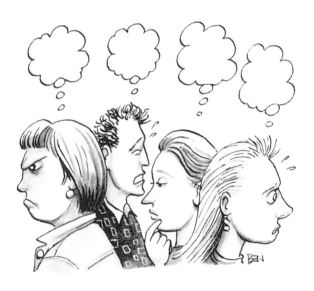

How does it feel
To be on your own
With no direction home
Like a complete unknown
Like a rolling stone?

Bob Dylan, 'Like a Rolling Stone'

It isn't easy to be a teenager. In the teenage years, a young woman is trying to establish her identity. She is trying to become relatively independent of her family, at the same time retaining her love and affection for her family. She is trying to relate to other people, increasingly intimately, as the years pass. She is likely to have some periods of elation and other periods when the world seems gloomy and when she feels unloved and unwanted. She is likely to go through periods when she behaves outrageously (as far as adults are concerned) as she tries to be part of her peer group. She might experiment with drugs. She might have problems at school that make her feel inadequate, unwanted, or rebellious.

In spite of the difficulties of adolescence, the majority of teenagers become adults without any severe psychological

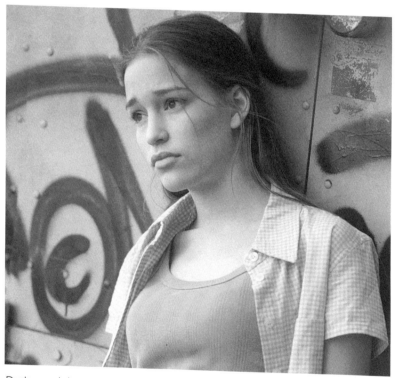

During adolescence, some teenagers experience bouts of depression or stress-related illnesses as they try to cope with the changes that are happening to them.

problems. How many teenagers do have psychological problems is difficult to determine, as in most cases a doctor or a psychologist is not consulted. Several attempts have been made to find the answer by inviting teenagers, chosen at random in a community, to fill in a questionnaire. Some of these investigations have surveyed only a small number of teenagers; others have been poorly organised. In the most recent and large survey of Australian women aged 13 to 17 years, 12 to 17 per cent were identified as having significant psychogical problems. These problems increase after a woman has had her first period and continue to rise throughout the teenage years. Four other good surveys, each studying more than 500 teenagers, have been made—one in Australia, one in Canada, and two in the UK. In these surveys, the researchers found that the most common psychological concerns expressed by teenagers were:

- difficulty in controlling their temper
- anxiety about their school work or about their job
- anxiety in social situations, around unfamiliar people
- difficulty concentrating
- frequent headaches or stomach pains
- feelings of hopelessness and sadness.

The surveys showed that during her teenage years one woman in six complained of one (and sometimes more) psychological upsets, which she or her doctors said were due to 'stress' or tension. Although most of the psychological problems seemed to have begun in the teenage years, in many cases the problem had existed since childhood and had become more obvious during adolescence.

Causes of psychological problems

A teenage woman is more likely to develop psychological problems if:

- Her parents don't get on with each other, and argue and bicker, or if their relationship is disturbed. The problems might continue whether the parents remain married, or separate.

- Her parents are always very critical of her, reject her, are hostile or brutal to her, or impose harsh discipline.
- Her parents are too busy to spare enough time for their daughter.
- Her parents have psychiatric problems or are criminals; they are poor role models.
- Her parents do not give their daughter the opportunity to talk with them, rejecting her attempts to communicate.
- Her family is large, poor, and lives in an unstable environment.

These families might be classed as 'problem' families, and both the parents and the teenagers might need help, although often they do not seek it. Only a few young women who are reared in these social conditions develop psychological problems.

Even in a close-knit, loving family, a teenager could develop psychological problems. These might occur because the teenager feels that she is not receiving the attention she believes she deserves or if her growing autonomy is not recognised. The problems might also occur because the teenage woman is angry about the way she perceives her parents treat her compared with the way she thinks other parents treat their daughters.

A more dramatic way in which a psychological upset could occur in the teenage years (as in all other years) is when a loved family member dies, or following the break-up of a close friendship with a girlfriend or a boyfriend.

In the school years, a teenage woman could develop psychological problems if she is not able to perform as well as her friends in school work or in sport, or is unpopular, bullied, or 'picked on' by her teachers. These feelings might lead to anxiety and feelings of panic. These feelings in turn might cause her to lose her appetite and prevent her from sleeping well, which makes her feel worse. She might play truant or refuse to go to school.

The psychological problems of being a teenager can also be increased if the teenager is unable to get a job after leaving school. Teenage unemployment has become increasingly common since the 1980s. Currently in most Western countries between 15 and 25 per cent of teenagers are unemployed or underemployed. Unemployment has adverse physical as well as psychological consequences. When a teenager is unable to obtain work, in spite of repeated attempts, she might feel she is a failure and that life is not worth living. Or she might become angry and aggressive to others, or to society in general, for not giving her a 'fair go'. Underemployment means that a person is able to obtain only a part-time job or a job that provides less stimulation or a lower status than she wants or is capable of. Like unemployment, underemployment can also lead to feelings of hopelessness, or the teenager might exhibit aggressive behaviour.

The psychological problems of unemployed and underemployed teenagers are aggravated if the teenager's family is not supportive and complain constantly about her appearance or lack of initiative.

Another reason some teenagers feel sad and hopeless is that the teenage years are a time of life when body image is very important. Teenage women are more likely than teenage men to feel less attractive physically. A teenage woman who is teased about her body shape could develop a poor self-image, feeling that she is unwanted and ugly. This perception might cause feelings of hopelessness. A study of more than 5000 teenagers in the USA found that if most females felt as 'good' about themselves and their body shape as did most males, they would be less likely to become unhappy and sad or feel hopeless.

Symptoms of psychological problems

About a quarter of adolescent girls complain of headaches that occur several times per week or even every day. There could be a medical reason for the headache, such as migraine, but in most cases they are caused by a stressful psychological problem that shows as a physical symptom. This is called somatisation. Another way the psychological upset shows itself is in pains in the abdomen that are not related to the woman's periods. One adolescent woman in seven complains of frequent abdominal pain. In nearly all cases, no physical cause is found. The pain is another example of somatisation.

A teenager who 'acts out' her frustrations by becoming a delinquent usually has had previous psychological upsets. She might vandalise property or steal, believing that she is paying back society and her family for their lack of concern for her needs. On the other hand, she might become sexually promiscuous and vent her frustrations by having casual sex with several partners in the hope that she will obtain gratification and perhaps status in her group. Such behaviour could result in an unwanted pregnancy or a sexually transmitted disease.

Some psychologists believe that more teenagers show aggressive behaviour today because they copy what they see on TV and in videos. The extent to which television affects a teenager's psychological well-being is considerable. In 1990, an expert committee of the American Academy of Pediatrics reported that they believed extensive television viewing was one cause of aggressive or violent behaviour, which might be sexual in nature. This type of behaviour was more common among teenage men, but also occurred among teenage women. The authors of the report based their claim on a study that showed that adolescents aged between 12 and 17 spent an average of twenty-three hours per week watching television or videos. In a twelve-month period TV programs had shown several thousand murders and more than 14,000 sexual references or innuendos. They speculated that watching violence on TV and in videos might cause some teenagers to 'act out' their psychological problems by aggressive or violent behaviour.

Psychological problems might cause a teenager to abuse alcohol and other drugs. In other words, the teenager might engage in risk-taking behaviour (this is considered in chapter 16). If the psychological disturbance is severe it can cause the teenager to become clinically depressed. Clinical depression is not just loneliness or unhappiness, which are common feelings during the teenage years, as they are at other times of life. Clinical depression is discussed later in this chapter.

Coping with psychological problems

Most teenagers do not develop severe psychological problems, although about 15 per cent do experience some psychological upsets. If a teenager feels she has a problem that is causing her distress, she might be helped if she learns to relax and gives herself time to relax.

There are several types of relaxation to choose from. Some people relax by taking exercise, or playing a game or sport that they enjoy. Some people relax by reading a book, becoming absorbed in the activities and behaviour of the characters.

Some people relax by watching television, although, as mentioned above, violence on television might not be conducive to relaxation. Some people relax by doing tai chi, yoga, or meditation.

Although these suggestions help many people to relax, they take time. Some people choose a simple relaxation exercise, which can be repeated several times a day without difficulty. It only takes a few minutes, and it will make you feel less tense. If possible, repeat the exercise four to six times per day. You can do this exercise by yourself or, if you prefer, join a group that teaches relaxation. This is how you do the exercise:

1 Sit in a comfortable chair, or lie down where you are unlikely to be disturbed for a few minutes.
2 Make sure you are comfortable, with your hands and legs uncrossed and with no tight clothing such as shoes or a belt.
3 Listen to the sounds around you, for example traffic outside, the clock in the room, the family in another room. If you are aware of these sounds they will not disturb you when you are relaxing.
4 Close your eyes. Although your eyelids might flicker, this will stop soon.
5 Become aware of your breathing.
6 Take a breath, and then let the rate of your breathing slow down so that it is about the same as when you are asleep. Don't try to force it. Just let it slow down so that it is comfortable.

7 Each time you breathe out, let your body relax so that you feel limp and floppy and warm and heavy as though you were sinking into the chair or a bed.

8 Keep thinking of your breathing, and keep it slowed down.

9 Think of your arm muscles, and let them relax. Then think of your leg muscles, then your body muscles, then your neck muscles, your face and forehead muscles; let each group of muscles relax so that you are completely relaxed.

10 Each time, spend no more than two minutes doing the exercise.

Unfortunately only 50 per cent of teenagers who have psychological problems seek help, and if they do it is usually from their school counsellor or family doctor. It is good to talk about problems, even if they do not seem as bad as other people's problems. Talking can help you to understand what is happening, what might occur in the future, and if there are things you or others can do that will provide relief.

Depression

Given the changes they are experiencing, it is not surprising that some teenagers become clinically depressed (although there are far fewer depressed teenagers than adults). Between the ages of 14 and 19, up to a quarter of teenage women will suffer a major depressive episode. Another way of looking at the problem is that between one and five of every hundred teenage girls are depressed at any one time, compared with about one teenage male in every hundred. Adolescence seems to be more difficult for young women than for young men. In 2000, a large survey suggested the number of young women suffering from depression was higher than 5 in 100.

Clinical depression is diagnosed when the person shows at least two of the following symptoms for two weeks or longer (based on the criteria developed by the American College of Psychiatrists). The person:

• loses interest or pleasure in all, or almost all, usually pleasurable happenings; in other words feels hopeless

- doesn't feel much better, even temporarily, when something good happens
- is usually sadder in the mornings
- keeps waking up early (at least two hours before she usually wakes up) and can't get to sleep again
- loses her appetite or starts overeating
- can't be bothered doing anything, feels tired, and has no energy
- finds it difficult to concentrate or make decisions.

If a teenage woman is feeling clinically depressed, a relaxation program is probably not enough to help her, and she might need to seek help from a sympathetic health professional (a doctor or a psychologist) who will listen while she talks about her feelings and problems.

Often the periods of depression alternate with episodes of anger. Anger might be expressed by assaulting others or by deliberately harming herself. An investigation in Melbourne found that one teenager in twenty had deliberately hurt herself or himself in the previous twelve months.

In severe cases the depression might lead the adolescent woman to attempt to commit suicide. Suicide becomes a more frequent problem in the later teenage years and is four times less common among adolescent females than among adolescent males. In Western countries, suicide is increasing as unemployment rates among young people grow. In many Western countries, between eight and sixteen adolescent men and between one and four adolescent women in every 100,000 commit suicide each year. Most people attempting suicide give warnings weeks or days before the attempt. They are seeking help and most want to be rescued. If a teenager feels suicidal, she should find someone who she can talk to about her problems. Help is at hand. Our society is now promoting community awareness of mental health and access to people who can help.

Chapter Sixteen
Risk-taking

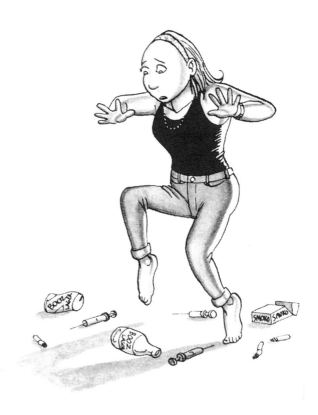

If you drink, then drive, you're a bloody idiot!
Traffic Accident Commission

Throughout recorded history, young people have been more likely to engage in risky forms of behaviour than older people, although the difference is not as marked as was once thought. Recent research suggests that teenagers are no more likely than adults to display impulsiveness or risk-taking behaviour or to be unable to understand the consequences of their acts.

In Western societies it is accepted that young people involve themselves in risky behaviour. They can rock-climb or bungee-jump, or engage in risky contact sports, but the risk is limited by training and by learning how to make the activity less risky. Other activities are inherently more risky and can cause damage to others. One such activity is driving a car fast and dangerously, particularly when affected by alcohol. Drug-taking can be safe or very risky. The remainder of this chapter is concerned with drugs.

Why do some teenagers start taking drugs?

Like most adults, teenagers take drugs. Some are legal drugs such as alcohol and tobacco; others are 'illegal' drugs, which include marijuana, ecstasy, hypnotics, cocaine, and heroin. Table 16.1 lists the percentages of young women in New South Wales who regularly use drugs.

One question that needs to be asked is: why do some teenagers use drugs? The answer is not clear, but some reasons have been found. First, teenagers start taking drugs, particularly the legal drugs, because drug-taking is regarded as socially acceptable among friends and others of the same age group, who put pressure on the teenager to conform to their views. In other words, they take drugs to feel 'cool' or to 'fit in'. Second, they take drugs out of curiosity and the need to experience new and novel experiences. Third, using legal drugs makes a teenager feel more grown-up and independent, particularly when she or he sees adults smoking and drinking. Fourth, if parents drink or smoke, their children are likely to copy them. Fifth, taking drugs (and this includes 'illegal' drugs) might make a difficult reality seem more acceptable, by blurring the pain, disappointment, and stresses of living. To most teenagers the present is more real and important than an uncertain future, so the long-term consequences of drugs, for example the increased chance of a smoker having a heart attack or lung cancer when middle-aged, is ignored.

Drug-taking usually follows a sequence. Alcohol and cigarettes are the first drugs taken, particularly when teenagers 'party'. During the party, having lost some degree of control by alcohol, a teenager will be offered marijuana by one of her friends. She smokes it and enjoys the feeling, but this does not mean that she will be hooked on marijuana. Twenty per cent of teenagers have tried marijuana, but fewer than 4 per cent use it weekly.

How common is drug-taking?

The proportion of young women in New South Wales, aged 14–19, who use various drugs is shown in table 16.1. The latest survey only reported adolescents aged 13 to 17 years. As you might expect, the older the teenager, the more likely she is to have taken drugs. The use of some drugs is increasing, as you can see if you look at table 16.1. Studies in the USA show similar

Table 16.1 Drugs used by young women aged 14–19 in New South Wales

Drug	1986 (%)	1989 (%)	1996 (%)	2000* (%)
Alcohol				
At least once per week	30	25	35	
In the last month				39
More than 5 drinks at least once in previous 2 weeks (heavy drinkers)	28	20	20	20
Tobacco				
Daily/occasionally	30	25	20	
In the last month				26
Marijuana				
Ever used	28	20	25	29
Used weekly	6	4	10	
In the last month				11

Analgesics				
Used more than 3 times in past month	34	42	12	8
Stimulants				
Obtained illegally (ever used)	9	7	6	6
Hallucinogens				
Ever used	5	3	6	4
Narcotics				
Heroin (ever used)	3	2	4	1
Designer drugs				
Ecstacy (ever used)				1

* Teenagers 13–17 years, National Survey of Mental Health and Wellbeing, Child and Adolescent Component 2000

Table 16.2 Standard drinks of different alcoholic beverages

	Beer		
	Superlight	*Light*	*Ordinary*
Strength	Approx. 0.9% by volume	Approx. 2–3% by volume	Approx. 4–5% by volume
Amount	5 middies (5 x 285 mL)	2 middies (2 x 285 mL)	1 middie (285 mL)
Alcohol content	10 gm	10 gm	10 gm

	Table wine	*Fortified wine*	*Spirits*
Strength	Approx. 10% by volume	Approx. 20% by volume	Approx. 40% by volume
Amount	1 glass (120 mL)	1 glass (60 mL)	1 nip (30 mL)
Alcohol content	10 gm	10 gm	10 gm

findings. The opportunity to use drugs has increased from 1995 to 1998; six additional young teenagers in every hundred had the opportunity to use marijuana and ecstacy. The use of ecstacy rose from 2 to 6.5% from 1995 to 1998 among teenagers aged 14 to 19 years. Most of this use is likely to be by 17 to 19 year olds.

Teenagers and alcohol

In 1984, Gerald Lundberg wrote: 'What we do in our society is to raise our kids until they are 10, 12 or 14. Then we toss them out into an ocean of alcohol and we don't give them swimming lessons. Some swim and some sink and we can't predict which will do which.'

A major problem is that in nearly all Western societies, alcohol is a socially acceptable drug. In one sense, alcohol is also a food, but a very poor food nutritionally as it contains no protein or vitamins and provides only energy. However, if the energy provided from alcohol is more than that needed for the

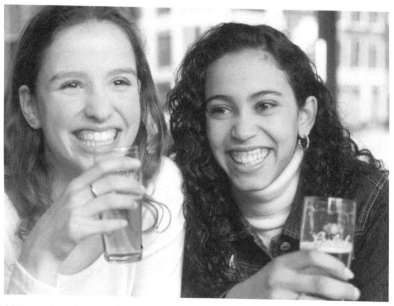

Many adults began drinking alcohol when they were teenagers.

body's functions, it is converted into fat (which explains the beer belly of some middle-aged men).

Pure alcohol is tasteless, but alcoholic drinks are made by mixing alcohol with other ingredients that provide taste and colour. The resulting alcoholic beverages have different tastes and colours, and have different alcoholic strengths. For example, beer contains between 0.9 per cent and 6.0 per cent alcohol, whereas table wines contain between 11 and 13 per cent alcohol and spirits between 37 and 40 per cent alcohol.

These variations in the amount of alcohol in 100 mL of a beverage have led to the concept of a 'standard drink'. A standard drink contains 10 grams of pure alcohol, and the concept enables comparisons of different volumes to be made. For example, a standard drink (also known as one unit of alcohol) of ordinary beer contains 12.5 mL (10 gm) of alcohol in the 285 mL drink. The relationship of the volume of different alcoholic drinks is shown in table 16.2. You can see that 285 mL of ordinary beer contains the same amount of alcohol as a 120 mL glass of table wine or 30 mL (a nip) of whisky.

Most moderate teenage drinkers usually drink only one kind of alcoholic beverage. More teenage men drink beer than wine or spirits, whereas more teenage women drink wine or premixed drinks than beer. But those who are heavy drinkers tend to mix their drinks, drinking spirits and liqueurs as well as their usual kind of drink.

Three-quarters of adults drink alcohol; some in moderation, some excessively. Many of these adults started drinking alcohol when they were teenagers. Fewer women than men drink alcohol. A survey in New South Wales found that one teenage woman in ten aged between 14 and 18 drank alcohol every day compared with one teenage man in seven. However, equivalent amounts of alcohol affect women more than men. This is because women's bodies do not deal with alcohol as well as men's bodies, partly because women have more fatty tissues to absorb the alcohol and less body fluid to dilute it. Alcohol does not need to be digested. It passes straight into the bloodstream, through the walls of the stomach and the intestine. In the blood it is carried to the liver and then around the body, being absorbed preferentially by fatty tissues, including the brain.

Effects of alcohol

The effects of alcohol on the body depend on the quantity of alcohol consumed and how fast it is consumed. The effects also depend on the weight of the person and the amount of fat in her or his body, whether the alcohol was consumed with food, and the person's mood. Different individuals can also tolerate alcohol differently.

- If your blood alcohol level is less than 0.05 per cent you feel good, your inhibitions are reduced, and you become relaxed and tend to talk a lot.
- If you drink more alcohol, so that your blood alcohol level is between 0.05 and 0.08 per cent, you become 'woozy', and your judgment and movements are affected.
- Higher levels of alcohol in your blood are dangerous. A blood level between 0.08 per cent and 0.15 per cent causes blurred vision and slurred speech. Your balance is affected and you stagger. You might feel sick and vomit. You might fall asleep and remember nothing of what happened when you got drunk.
- If you drink still more, so that your blood alcohol level is between 0.2 and 0.5 per cent, you are dead drunk, stuporous and snoring, your mouth dribbling. You will remember nothing of the episode. And if your blood alcohol level exceeds 0.45 per cent you need your stomach pumped; otherwise you might die from alcohol poisoning.

You can estimate the amount of alcohol in your blood by doing a complicated calculation, but if you are drinking you are unlikely to be able, or want, to do the maths! An easy approximation is that if you weigh between 30 and 49 kg, and you drink more than one standard drink an hour, your blood alcohol level will exceed 0.05 per cent. If you weigh between 50 and 70 kg, you can drink two standard drinks before your blood level exceeds 0.05 per cent.

Moderate drinking

The Bible says that a little alcohol may be 'good for thy stomach's sake'. This was very perceptive of the writer, because it has been shown recently that a small amount of alcohol taken regularly can, to some extent, protect a middle-aged person from a heart attack.

It follows that a moderate amount of alcohol, that is, no more than two standard drinks up to four times per week, will do a healthy, non-pregnant woman no harm. The only danger is that by drinking more than two standard drinks at a party or at dinner, you might increase your blood alcohol level to more than 0.05 and then drive home. If you are caught by the police and breathalysed you will probably be in trouble.

Heavy drinking

Heavy drinking, on the other hand, is dangerous to your health and might be dangerous to others if you become violent or drive when drunk. Heavy drinking, that is, drinking more than twenty-eight standard drinks per week if you are male and more than fourteen drinks per week if you are female, is not common among teenage women, but it does occur. Heavy drinking can occur in binge-drinking or in drinking every day. Studies in Newcastle (New South Wales) and Adelaide (South Australia) in 1991 found that 9 to 11 per cent of young women aged between 15 and 24 were heavy drinkers.

Teenage heavy drinkers are more likely to be delinquent than moderate drinkers or abstainers. They often binge-drink until they are inebriated, and drinking often causes them to get into trouble.

Alcohol abuse and your health

If you drink heavily for a number of years it becomes dangerous to your health (see figure 16.1) and costly to the community. One adult in every six is a heavy drinker, and more men (14 per cent) than women (8 per cent) drink heavily. The abuse of alcohol in terms of medical care, lost work, accidents, and crime costs the United States more than $70 billion each year.

The dangers of heavy drinking do not become apparent at once, and different people are affected differently. Alcohol can damage every body system, but those most often affected are the liver and the brain. Alcohol abuse leads to liver damage in six out of every ten heavy drinkers, and in two of them the damage is severe, causing cirrhosis of the liver. Female heavy drinkers are more likely to develop cirrhosis than are men. Since the 1960s, alcohol-induced liver cirrhosis has become the fourth most common cause of death among men older than 30 and the eighth in women of the same age. As more women now drink heavily than used to be the case, the difference is being reduced.

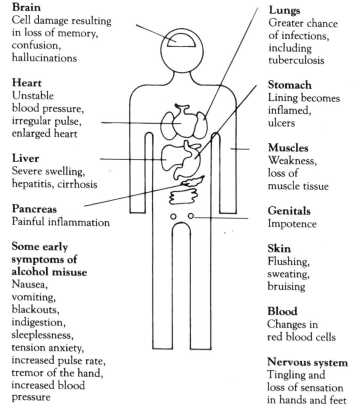

Brain
Cell damage resulting in loss of memory, confusion, hallucinations

Heart
Unstable blood pressure, irregular pulse, enlarged heart

Liver
Severe swelling, hepatitis, cirrhosis

Pancreas
Painful inflammation

Some early symptoms of alcohol misuse
Nausea, vomiting, blackouts, indigestion, sleeplessness, tension anxiety, increased pulse rate, tremor of the hand, increased blood pressure

Lungs
Greater chance of infections, including tuberculosis

Stomach
Lining becomes inflamed, ulcers

Muscles
Weakness, loss of muscle tissue

Genitals
Impotence

Skin
Flushing, sweating, bruising

Blood
Changes in red blood cells

Nervous system
Tingling and loss of sensation in hands and feet

Figure 16.1 The effects of alcohol on the body. Repeated excessive drinking will affect these organs and tissues in the long term.

The brain is affected by alcohol abuse only slightly less frequently than the liver. An alcoholic's memory deteriorates, she is unable to grasp new ideas and might develop bizarre jealousies or hatreds. In family situations this can lead to irrational behaviour, to quarrels, and to physical abuse. If an alcoholic parent has children, his or her behaviour might so affect the child that her school work deteriorates or she escapes from an intolerable home environment.

Do I have a drinking problem?

You can tell whether you have a drinking problem by completing the questionnaire below. If you score up to two Bs you are a sensible drinker. If you score three or four Bs, take care and try to make a few changes. If you score between five and seven Bs, you are heading for a drinking problem.

Alcohol and driving

Many young people enjoy driving because it represents freedom and independence, a feeling of being grown-up. Many like the excitement of driving fast; they also like to drink. By the age of 20, one Australian teenager in six is a 'hazardous drinker', consuming more than 140 gm of alcohol per week. If a teenager (or anyone) drinks large quantities of alcohol and then drives a car, the results can be horrific. Car crashes can cause both minor and severe injuries and/or death to anyone involved in an accident, regardless of who caused the accident and whether a person is a driver or a passenger. Young people aged between 17 and 24 are at greatest risk of any age group of dying or being injured in a car crash. They are at more than three times the risk of dying than the next age group (those aged 25–34). Each year, one person in every 1200 aged between 17 and 24 dies as a result of a car crash, compared with one person in every 4500 in the next age group. Although young men are at four times the risk of young women, clearly there is still a significant chance that a young woman will be involved in a car accident.

Each year, one in thirty young men aged between 17 and 21 will be seriously injured in a car crash and require admission to hospital. Not all of these car crashes will be caused by drunk drivers, but many will.

Am I a sensible drinker?

•	Do I find it difficult to refuse alcohol?	Yes B	No A
•	Can I enjoy a day without alcohol?	Yes A	No B
•	Do I know how much alcohol I drink each week?	Yes A	No B
•	Do I drink alcohol before driving?	Yes B	No A
•	Is alcohol spoiling my sport?	Yes B	No A
•	Has anyone in my family or my friends ever made comments against my drinking?	Yes B	No A
•	Do I drink with 'sensible' limits?	Yes A	No B

Sobering up

Most of the alcohol that you drink is broken down in your liver. The liver can break down the alcohol only at a fixed rate and is able to metabolise (get rid of) about 10 gm of alcohol—one standard drink—per hour. Nothing can speed up the rate at which alcohol is metabolised—not black coffee, exercise, vomiting, or cold showers. Drinking coffee or having a shower might help you to feel more awake and less dopey, but it won't lower your blood alcohol level.

Pregnancy and alcohol

If you become pregnant it is wise not to drink any alcohol, and certainly no more than one standard drink, occasionally, as alcohol can damage your baby. Heavy drinking can lead to a baby with fetal alcohol syndrome. Babies with fetal alcohol syndrome grow slowly, both before and after birth, and are often mentally retarded.

Prevention of alcohol abuse

Of all the so-called drugs of abuse, alcohol is the most frequently abused ... and alcohol remains the cause of the greatest number of health and social problems.

Director-General, World Health Organization

Can someone who enjoys moderate drinking be helped to avoid becoming a heavy drinker and so avoid these problems? Education programs about the problems of drinking alcohol have been tried often, but their effectiveness has been limited. That is not to say that knowledge about the effects of alcohol is not useful, but it does not seem to deter some people from drinking heavily. It appears that the most effective measures in reducing alcohol-related problems are: (1) limiting the number of outlets from which alcoholic beverages can be obtained; and (2) raising the price of alcoholic drinks.

Teenagers and tobacco

It is said that Columbus discovered America and, in return, brought syphilis and tobacco back to Europe. Tobacco, usually smoked in the form of cigarettes, is our second most used drug, although the number of smokers is declining. For example, in 1945, 72 per cent of men and 26 per cent of women were smokers. Forty years later, in 1985, 30 per cent of men and 27 per cent of women smoked.

The decline in smoking also occurred among teenagers. Surveys in New South Wales show that between 1983 and 1988 the number of teenagers aged between 12 and 16 who smoked dropped by 6 per cent. In 1989, 13 per cent of teenage men and 17 per cent of teenage women were regular smokers. However, the number of teenage women smokers is rising again.

Why do teenagers smoke? Some start because their parents smoke and smoking is acceptable in their home. Some start smoking because their friends smoke, and they do not wish to stand out as non-smokers. It is not clear why more teenage women than teenage men smoke. It might be because teenage women feel that it is sophisticated to smoke and they believe that if they smoke they will not gain weight.

Teenage smoking—the facts

More teenage girls smoked in the 1990s than in the 1980s, but boys who smoke generally smoke more heavily than girls. A quarter of teenagers are smokers, most starting between the ages of 12 and 16. Nearly all habitual smokers started the habit during adolescence. Teenagers smoke because:

- their best friend or peers smoke
- of the glamorous advertising of cigarettes
- their parents smoke
- they believe that they will not gain weight and might lose weight
- they believe that smoking signifies maturity, control, defiance, and a means of coping with stress.

However, smokers tend to be rebellious, have a poor self-image, and indulge in other forms of risk-taking behaviour.

Effects of smoking tobacco

When smoked, tobacco releases nicotine, tar, carbon monoxide gas, and about 4000 other chemicals. Nicotine is a poison. Three drops of pure nicotine would kill an adult. For this reason, cigarette manufacturers limit the nicotine content of a cigarette to 1.4 mg—a safe dose. Nicotine causes bodily changes. At first it stimulates the brain and, about half an hour later, produces a relaxed feeling. It increases the heart rate, causes a rise in blood pressure, and reduces the circulation in some blood vessels. This is why regular smoking of cigarettes increases the possibility of a heart attack in middle age.

The tar released from cigarettes, in the form of particles in the inhaled smoke, is a cause of lung cancer and other respiratory diseases. It makes the air sacs in the lungs less flexible, which can cause smoker's cough, wheezing, and shortness of breath. A person of average size who smokes one packet of cigarettes per day inhales about half a cupful of tar over a year.

The inhaled carbon monoxide gas reduces the amount of oxygen that the lungs can pass to the blood, so the tissues receive less oxygen.

Smoking is a health hazard
Long-term smoking leads to:
- shortness of breath, an increased risk of chest infections, and lung damage (emphysema)
- narrowing and hardening of the arteries, particularly in the heart and the legs
- an increased risk of a heart attack
- an increased risk of cancer of the mouth, the larynx, and the bladder
- an increased risk of cancer of the uterine cervix in women
- an increased risk of lung cancer in both sexes
- an increased chance of dry skin and wrinkles as smoking accelerates the physical signs of ageing
- an increased risk of giving birth to a growth-retarded baby.

In spite of these known risks, most teenage smokers do not perceive them as relevant as they are so remote from their lives.

Passive smoking

Smoking not only affects the smoker but might also damage the health of others who inhale the smoker's smoke. Second-hand smoke is the smoke breathed out by the smoker and in by the passive smoker. Sidestream smoke is the smoke from the burning end of the cigarette which the person breathes in. This smoke has more inhaled tobacco poisons than mainstream smoke.

Passive smoking is now believed to increase asthma and respiratory complaints, and might reduce the weight of an unborn baby.

Smoking and pregnancy

If you are a smoker, pregnancy is a good time to quit or, if you can't, to cut down your cigarettes to fewer than ten per day. Women who smoke are likely to have a baby who weighs about 8 per cent less at birth than a baby of a non-smoker. This is because the inhaled tar and carbon monoxide gas cut down the amount of oxygen and nutrients reaching the fetus, preventing the fetus from growing properly.

Giving up smoking

Giving up smoking is difficult. It is much easier not to start smoking than to give it up. Smoking is addictive, and most smokers become dependent on cigarettes, which means that smoking becomes central to the person's thoughts, emotions, and activities. That is why it is difficult to quit smoking.

Research has shown that nearly 80 per cent of smokers began smoking in their teens. A person in her twenties who has never smoked is unlikely to start smoking and become an addict. More than 90 per cent of smokers have wanted to quit when they learn about the dangers of smoking to their health, but few have succeeded: only 3 per cent of smokers successfully quit each year. There are several reasons for this. First, as tobacco smoking is addictive, you continue to feel that you must have a cigarette. And if you do not continue smoking you might get withdrawal symptoms when you stop or cut down your nicotine intake. You might feel nervous and tense, not sleep well, lose concentration, develop headaches, or start eating more. Many smokers know that if you quit smoking you are likely to put on weight, something young women desperately want to avoid.

As quitting is so hard, and so often unsuccessful, it is better not to start. But if you are a smoker you can quit. You will find it is worth it. You will feel better, and your health will improve.

How to quit smoking

The first step is to decide to quit smoking. Most smokers make this decision several times before they quit for life. Some people find it easier to go 'cold turkey'—to stop suddenly—than to cut down gradually. If you do choose to cut down gradually, you should make a firm date for quitting, not more than two weeks away.

Some people find that they need help to quit. They can obtain this support if they join an anti-smoking group, seek help from a psychologist, or obtain some sort of 'quit pack' from their doctor or an anti-smoking organisation.

Teenagers and illegal drugs

This section discusses marijuana, cocaine, and heroin. Some teenagers take mild tranquillisers, such as Rohypnol and Mogadon (which are not illegal if prescribed by a doctor), a growing number use ecstasy, and a tiny number have access to LSD (lysergic acid), angel dust, magic mushrooms, and mescaline, but any teenager who needs information about the dangers of these drugs should contact the various drug and alcohol information services available in their city, state, or country.

Certain matters are common to all the illegal drugs. First, the effects of the drug depend on:
- how much of the drug is taken
- the way the drug is taken
- the person's size, weight, and health
- the person's mood
- the person's experience with the drug, in other words, the person's tolerance of the drug (so that more and more is needed to achieve the same effect), and the person's dependence on the drug.

Second, withdrawal symptoms occur if a person who is dependent on the drug decides to stop using or reduces the amount used. The withdrawal symptoms can be severe and very distressing, sometimes painful enough to lead to suicide. Therefore anyone withdrawing from any drug should contact their local community health centre or a doctor for help and support.

Marijuana

Marijuana (grass or dope) and hashish come from the cannabis plant. Marijuana is made from the dried flowers and leaves of the plant, and is usually smoked in hand-rolled cigarettes, called joints, or in water pipes called bongs.

Hashish is made from the resin of the cannabis plant. The resin is dried and pressed into small blocks. Hashish is sold in small, light brown or black pieces, and is either mixed with tobacco and smoked or eaten in food. Hashish is stronger than marijuana and produces a greater effect.

More than a third of young people have tried marijuana at some time, but most do not use it often. Regular marijuana smokers also tend to smoke cigarettes and drink alcoholic beverages.

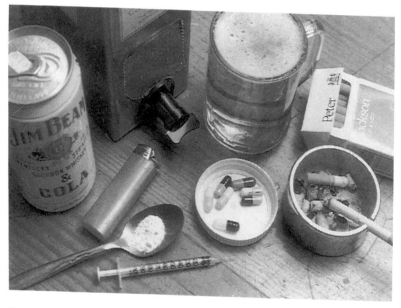

Drugs come in all different shapes and sizes, some legal, others illegal.

This practice could be dangerous as these drugs can intensify the effects of marijuana, often in unpredictable ways.

Effects of marijuana

People who use marijuana in small doses 'get high'. They lose their inhibitions, talk, and laugh a lot; they feel excited and might lose concentration. Their eyes become reddened, and their pulse rate goes up. The effects last for an hour or two and are followed by sleepiness and, often, a calm feeling. Marijuana used in large doses makes these effects stronger and longer lasting. Large doses can also produce confusion, restlessness, and changes in the perception of time, sound, and colour, or even hallucinations. Driving a car when high on marijuana is dangerous. Regular use of marijuana has been reported to cause loss of memory and reduction in concentration; paranoia; depression; and lack of motivation, so that performance at school or at work might suffer. In a few young people it may trigger an episode of schizophrenia or psychosis and predispose other young people to depression in later life.

Cocaine and crack

Cocaine is derived from the leaves of the coca plant by treating them with chemicals. This produces a white powder, which users inhale through the nose. People who sell cocaine often dilute the powder with powdered milk, bleach, or sugar in order to increase their profits. Crack is a very pure type of cocaine and is sold in the form of small crystals or 'rocks'. It is usually smoked. Crack is now a major drug problem in the USA, and has appeared in the UK and Australia.

Effects of cocaine

As with the other drugs, the effects of cocaine depend on how much of the drug is taken, the size and weight of the person, whether it is taken alone or in combination with other drugs, and the mood of the person. A single, low dose of cocaine causes a feeling of well-being, increased alertness, and energy. It causes agitation and sexual arousal but also unpredictable or violent behaviour. Larger doses increase the chance that the person will engage in violent behaviour, will be restless, experience headaches and dizziness, lose concentration, and lose interest in sex. Withdrawal symptoms include: severe depression, suicidal feelings, shaking fits, vomiting, hunger, disturbed sleep, and a craving for cocaine.

New designer drugs

Ecstacy is one of the new synthetic designer drugs being produced. These drugs are like amphetamines (which are in fact old drugs that are still popular and currently used) in chemical structure and biological actions. Ecstasy is a 'party drug' and easily obtained (not always pure; see Heroin) around night clubs and at all night 'raves'; it makes you feel full of energy, very sociable and aroused sexually, and able to continue dancing all night. Contrary to early beliefs these drugs are not safe even when taken in the short-term; the toxic dose can be the same as the recreational dose. Deaths have been associated with elevated body temperature, dehydration, breakdown of muscle cells, and elevated heart rate and blood pressure leading to heart failure. Depression, fatigue, anxiety, panic attacks, and difficulty concentrating can be present for two to three days following use; this will effect school and work performance. Brief psychotic episodes and hallucinations usually, but not always, cease when the drug wears off.

Heroin

Heroin (also called smack, junk, or horse) is a very powerful and addictive drug. It is one of the drugs that are obtained from the seed pods of the opium poppy. These drugs include opium, morphine (from which heroin is manufactured), and codeine. These drugs are pain-killers and pure heroin is the most powerful. Street heroin is rarely pure. It is usually mixed with other substances, such as sugar, talcum powder, or cheaper drugs such as amphetamines, so that the dealer's profit is higher.

Effects of heroin

Heroin is injected into a blood vessel. At first it acts on the brain so that the user has a rush—a feeling of well-being. Quite quickly this feeling passes and is succeeded by a feeling of warmth and drowsiness. The user hardly feels any pain or hunger, and his or her sexual urge diminishes.

Heroin is addictive. This means that you can become dependent on the drug very quickly, often within a few days of use. When you become dependent, heroin becomes central to all your thoughts, emotions, and activities. You have to have another fix, no matter what. You can't stop using the drug or even reduce the amount you use. You have become physically dependent on heroin, and your body needs it to function normally. Heroin damages your health, and there is a chance you will die from an overdose. Many heroin users share needles and syringes, and this is one way in which hepatitis and HIV (the virus causing AIDS) spread. You might develop abscesses, collapsed veins, or respiratory diseases or become severely constipated. Withdrawal symptoms begin a few hours after the last fix. They include restlessness, a runny nose and eyes, stomach and leg cramps, diarrhoea, goosebumps, and an intense craving for heroin.

Heroin and pregnancy

Heroin affects the health of the unborn baby. During the pregnancy the baby's growth is poor, partly because the mother is often unable to afford nutritious food because of her dependence and is undernourished, and partly because heroin crosses the placenta, so the baby becomes dependent on heroin. After birth, the baby develops severe withdrawal symptoms and needs extra care. This is recognised by health authorities, and special units have been established in some hospitals to care for heroin-dependent pregnant women and their babies.

How do you break your addiction?

It is often not recognised that only a few teenagers use heroin. Fewer than one teenager in every 2000 is dependent on heroin.

But if you are dependent, and want to break the habit, help is available. The programs developed by the drug and alcohol authorities, including counselling and the methadone program, can help dependent people through a difficult and traumatic time. As with any drug of addiction, however, it is easier and better not to begin than to try to quit.

Appendix

A map of the reproductive world

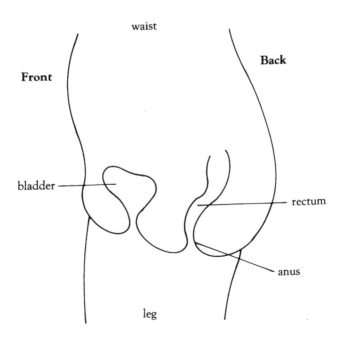

Figure 1 Try to draw in where you think your vagina, uterus, and ovaries are, and how big they are in relation to the rest of your body.

When you go to a new city and want to explore it, it is advisable to buy a map, so that you can find out where you are, what you want to see, and how to get there. When you explore the outside of your body you can see what it looks like, but the inside of your body is hidden and mysterious. And no part of the body is more mysterious than the genital organs of a woman. The mystery is maintained because many people are embarrassed to talk openly about such parts of the body as the *pudenda*, the vulva, the vagina, the uterus, the Fallopian tubes, and the ovaries. Even one of the medical names for the woman's external genital organs, the pudenda, is a derogatory word: it derives from the Latin word meaning 'shameful'. To many people it is shameful to talk of the genital organs and even more shameful to explore them. But if a woman is to understand her body she needs a map, so that she can understand what is attached to what, how the organs are related to each other, and how they function.

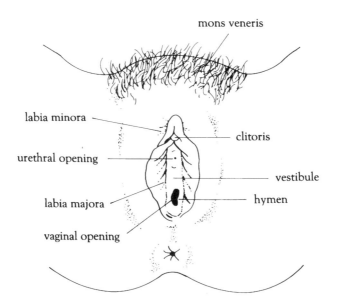

Figure 2   The external genitals of a virgin, seen from between the legs.

Unlike the genital organs of the male, most of the female genital organs lie deep within the woman's bony pelvis, hidden from view. This makes them mysterious, and many teenagers have no idea of what the uterus is like, where it is in the pelvis, and how big it is. Perhaps you would like to try an experiment. Using your memory of earlier chapters in this book, draw on figure 1 on page 262 where you think your vagina, uterus, and ovaries are. Then compare your ideas with the reality shown in the next few pages.

A good way to start to find your way around your genital anatomy is to have a look. Start by standing in front of a long mirror. You will observe that the lower part of your abdomen is covered with hair. But you can't see your genital organs because they are hidden. To look at those organs that are on the surface of your body, lie on your back, relax and be comfortable, with a few pillows beneath your head. Draw up your legs and open them, and look 'down there' using a hand mirror. This is what you will see (see figure 2).

The external genital organs

The anatomical name for the external genitals is the *vulva*. It is made up of several structures that surround the entrance to the vagina, each of which has its own separate function. The *labia majora* (the large lips of the vagina) are two large folds of skin that contain sweat glands and hair follicles embedded in fat. The size of the labia majora varies considerably with age. In infancy and in old age they are small, and the fat is not present; in the reproductive years between puberty and the menopause, they are well filled with fatty tissue. In front (looked at from between your legs), they join together in the pad of fat that lies over the pelvic bone and is called the mount of Venus (*mons veneris*). Both of the labia, and more particularly the mons veneris, are covered with hair, the quantity of which varies from woman to woman. But if you look, and separate your labia, you will notice that there is little or no hair on their inner side.

The pubic hair on your abdomen usually ends in a straight line so that it is triangular in appearance, as you will have noticed when you looked at yourself in front of a mirror. The amount of hair varies. Some women have a lot of pubic hair, some have only scanty pubic hair. Most women have springy, curly hair. If your family came from southern Europe the pubic hair might not look triangular but extend up towards your navel (belly button). If your family came from China you are likely to have scanty pubic hair. The amount of hair does not relate to your femininity or to how you will feel sexually. But if you feel that you are hairier than the other members of your family, you might like to visit a doctor to be reassured that your hormone levels are normal.

The *labia minora* (the small lips of the vagina) are delicate folds of skin that contain little fatty tissue. They vary in size and in front split into two folds, one of which passes over, and the other under, the clitoris. They are hairless. This part of the vaginal entrance often tears during childbirth. In the reproductive years the labia minora are partly hidden by the labia majora, but in childhood and old age the labia minora appear more prominent because the labia majora are relatively small. The actual size of the labia minora varies considerably between women. This is normal. Women in some African tribes have enormous labia minora that hang down between their legs like small curtains. From early childhood onwards, mothers stretch their daughters' labia minora because it is considered sexy to have long labia minora.

The *clitoris* lies in a fold of the inner lips of the vulva, in front of the pubic bone. Its size varies considerably, but it is usually that of a green pea. It is about 2 cm (3–4 inches) in length and becomes erect on sexual stimulation. Most of the clitoris can be felt only if it is pressed against the pubic bone, but its tip (or glans) is visible under the labial fold, which is also called the clitoral hood. The clitoris has the same origin in the embryo as the penis, which, in many ways, is the male equivalent. It has a rich supply of nerves, and is made up of spongy tissue that fills with blood on stimulation so that it enlarges. Stimulation of the clitoris, either indirectly during sexual intercourse or directly by gently stroking the clitoral area by finger or tongue, increases a woman's sexual arousal. Many women who do not reach orgasm during sexual intercourse do so easily and enjoyably by self-stimulation of the clitoris, or if their partner stimulates the clitoris using a finger or the tongue. In sexual intercourse, the movement of the man's penis in the vagina also stimulates the clitoris and can lead to the woman having an orgasm. As sexual excitement mounts, the clitoris increases in size.

The cleft below the clitoris and between the labia minora is called the *vestibule* (or entrance). Just below the clitoris is the external opening of the *urethra*, the part of the urinary tract that connects the bladder to the outside. Many women have no idea where their urethra opens into their external genitals. If you look, using your hand mirror, you should see your urethra as a dimple lying below your clitoris and above the entrance to your vagina. A few women find it hard to identify the dimple. If you are in doubt, put a pad beneath you and try to pass a small amount of urine. You will see the urine coming out of the urethra.

Behind the external urethral orifice is the hymen, which surrounds the vaginal orifice. The hymen is a thin fold of tissue with one or more holes in it (see figure 3). It varies considerably in shape and elasticity, but is generally stretched or torn during the first attempt at sexual intercourse. The tearing is usually followed by a small amount of bleeding. In many countries the rupture of the hymen (also called the maidenhead), and the consequent bleeding, was considered a sign that the woman was a

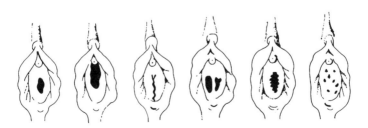

Figure 3 Different types of hymen.

virgin at the time of marriage, and the bed was inspected for evidence of blood on the morning after the first night of the honeymoon. Although an 'intact' hymen is considered a sign of virginity, it is not a reliable sign, as in some cases sexual intercourse fails to cause a tear, and in others the hymen might have been stretched previously by exploring fingers, either of the woman herself or of her sexual partner. The hymen can also be stretched by such activities as cycling or horse-riding. The stretching and tearing of the hymen at the first intercourse can be painful, particularly if the partners are apprehensive or ignorant of sexual matters. If the couple are relaxed with each other, the discomfort is minimal. Childbirth causes a much greater tearing of the hymen, and after delivery only a few tags remain. Some women feel these small tags and become anxious that they might be small growths.

Just outside the hymen, still within the entrance to your genitals but deep beneath the skin, are two collections of erectile tissues, which fill with blood during sexual arousal. Deep in the backward part of the vestibule are two pea-sized glands that also secrete mucus during sexual arousal and moisten the entrance to the vagina, so that the penis can enter it without discomfort. They are known as Bartholin's glands.

The part of the vulva between the vaginal entrance and the anus, and the muscles under the skin, form a pyramid-shaped wedge of tissue separating the vagina and the rectum. It is called the perineum. It is of considerable importance in childbirth as the muscles have to stretch to enable the baby to be born. In many cases the tissues tear, or a cut (called an episiotomy) is made to prevent tearing.

The internal genital organs

As these organs are inside your body they can't be seen, but if you feel comfortable about it, you can put one or two fingers in your vagina and at least feel what it is like. Far inside your vagina you will be able to feel your cervix, which projects like a

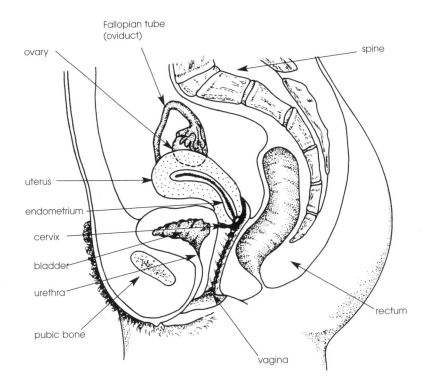

Figure 4 Internal genital organs (side view).

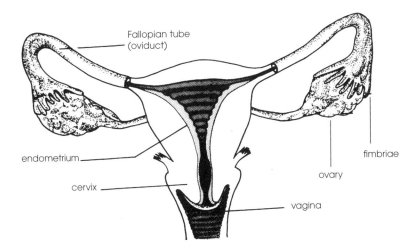

Figure 5 Internal genital organs (front view).

knob into the vagina and is smooth, rather like the tip of your nose but softer. The internal genital organs consist of the vagina, the uterus, the Fallopian tubes (or oviducts), and the ovaries (see figures 4 and 5).

The vagina is a muscular tube that stretches upwards and backwards from the vestibule to the uterus. As well as being muscular, it contains a well-developed network of veins, which become distended in sexual arousal. Normally the walls of the vagina lie close together. This means that the vagina is not the hollow tube many people believe it to be. However, the walls separate easily if a tampon is used during menstruation. They are easily parted by the penis at intercourse and, during child-birth, the vagina has to stretch very considerably to permit the baby to be born. In other words, it can stretch and take the shape of whatever is inside it. The vagina is about 9 cm (31–2 inches) long, and at the upper end the cervix (or neck) of the uterus projects into it. The vagina lies between the bladder in front and the rectum (or back passage) behind. At the sides it is surrounded and protected by the strong muscles of the floor of the pelvis. Unless the vagina has been damaged, injured, or tightened as a result of surgery, or has not developed due to an absence of sex hormones, its size is quite adequate for sexual intercourse. The woman who menstruates has a normal vagina. If she has difficulty at intercourse it might be due to inadequate sexual arousal, or because the woman hasn't relaxed the mus-cles that surround the vagina: it is not due to a small vagina.

The vagina also keeps itself clean. The walls of the vagina are formed by cells that lie on each other in layers twenty cells deep, like the bricks of a house wall. In the reproductive years, the top layer of cells is constantly being shed into the vagina. There, a small bacillus, which normally lives in the vagina, acts on the discarded cells to produce lactic acid. The lactic acid kills any contaminating germs that happen to get into the vagina. In other words, the vagina is self-cleansing.

In childhood the wall of the vagina is thin, and the produc-tion of lactic acid does not take place. From puberty onwards, at least until the menopause, the vagina is kept constantly moist by fluid that seeps through its walls. This fluid, the shed vaginal cells, and the lactic acid produce a small amount of whitish secretion. This is normal. If you are under stress, or anxious, or for several other reasons, the amount increases, as it does when you become sexually aroused. If the amount of the white discharge becomes heavy, or if it begins to be itchy, you should see a doctor, as you might have a vaginal infection (see chapter 14).

In old age the lining of the vagina becomes thin again and few cells are shed. This means little or no lactic acid is formed and contaminating germs can grow, which sometimes results in inflammation of the vagina.

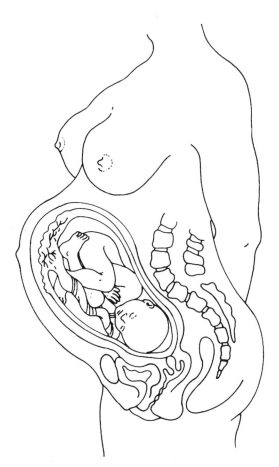

Figure 6   Pregnancy at forty weeks (just before birth).

The *uterus* (or womb) is a hollow muscular organ that averages 9 cm (31–2 inches) in length, 6 cm (21–2 inches) in width at its widest point, and weighs 100 gm (31–2 oz). You can see that it resembles a pear hung upside down. In pregnancy the uterus enlarges to weigh 1000 gm (2.2 lb), and is able to contain a baby measuring 40 cm (16 inches) in length (see figure 6). It is able to undergo these changes because of the complex structure of its muscle and its exceptional response to the female sex hormones.

The uterus is located in the middle of the bony pelvis, lying between the bladder in front and the bowel behind. It is pear-shaped, and its muscular front and back walls bulge into the cavity. This means that the uterus is nearly all muscle. Until pregnancy occurs, the cavity is normally narrow and slit-like, and viewed from the front it is triangular. The uterus is lined with a special tissue made up of glands in a network of cells. This tissue is called the *endometrium*, and it undergoes changes during each menstrual cycle.

Most of the endometrium, together with the blood and tissue fluid, is expelled when you have a menstrual period. Immediately it starts growing again, and the lining is quickly rebuilt. For descriptive purposes the uterus is divided into an upper part (or body) and a lower part (or *cervix uteri*: the neck of the uterus). The cervix projects into the upper part of the vagina. This is what you feel if you put a finger deep into your vagina. The cavity of the uterus narrows in the cervix, where it is called the cervical canal; it is widest in the body of the uterus, and then narrows again towards the cornu (or horn), where the cavity continues, finally becoming the hollow of the Fallopian tube.

The lower part of the uterus and the upper part of the cervix are supported by a sling of special tissues, called the cardinal ligament, which are attached to the muscles of the pelvic wall like a fan. Sometimes after childbirth these supports stretch and the uterus falls (or prolapses) down the vagina. If this occurs the cervix can be seen at the vaginal entrance when the woman strains down, for example in opening her bowels.

Normally the uterus lies bent forwards at an angle of 90 degrees to the vagina, resting on the bladder. As the bladder fills, it rotates backwards; as it empties, the uterus falls forward. In about 10 per cent of women the uterus lies bent backwards. This is called *retroversion*. Until a few years ago doctors believed that a retroverted uterus caused backache, pelvic pain, infertility, headache, constipation, and several other problems. They devised a variety of operations to 'correct' retroversion. Quite often the patient felt better—for a while. Doctors have now learnt that unless the retroverted uterus is 'fixed' backwards it causes no problems.

The *Fallopian tubes* (or oviducts) are two small, hollow tubes that stretch for about 10 cm (4 inches) from the upper part of the uterus, one on each side, to lie in contact with the ovary. Perhaps 'hollow' is the wrong word, as for most of its length the inner passage is only as big as a bristle on a hairbrush. The passage is surrounded by a muscle, which makes the outside of the Fallopian tube as large as a plastic drinking straw. The outer end of each Fallopian tube is divided into the long finger-like *fimbriae*, and it is thought that these sweep up the egg when it is expelled from the ovary. The tube is lined with cells shaped like goblets, which lie between cells with frond-like borders. The Fallopian tube is of great importance, as this is where fertilisation of the egg takes place, and it is likely that its secretions help to nourish the fertilised egg as it is transported towards the uterus by the wafting movements of the fronds.

The ovaries (or gonads) are two ovoid-shaped organs averaging 3.5 cm (11–2 inches) in length and 2 cm (3–4 inches) in width. In an infant they are small, delicate, thin structures, but after puberty they enlarge to reach full size. After the menopause they become small and wrinkled, and in old age are less than half their mature adult size. Each ovary has a centre made up of small cells and a mesh of vessels. Surrounding the centre is the ovary proper (the *cortex*) containing about 200,000 egg cells (*ova*), which lie in a cellular bed (the *stroma*). The egg cells and the stroma are protected by a thickened layer of tissue. In addition to containing egg cells on which all human life depends, the ovaries are also a hormone factory, producing the oestrogen and progesterone that are so important in making you a woman. The testes are the male equivalent.

Glossary

abortion *induced*: intentional termination of pregnancy; *spontaneous*: miscarriage.

acne often unsightly skin condition resulting from increased production of grease by skin glands; pimples.

addiction the inability to stop using a substance although you know it has (or might have) harmful effects on your body.

adolescence the period of time from puberty to adulthood.

AIDS (short for Acquired Immune Deficiency Syndrome) a sexually transmitted disease in which an affected person's immunity to infections is drastically reduced; usually fatal.

amenorrhoea the abnormal cessation of menstrual periods.

anaemia a lack of iron in the red blood cells, which might affect a person's health.

anorexia nervosa an illness affecting about one teenage woman in every hundred. The woman has a fear of becoming fat and starves herself. This leads to her becoming extremely thin and ceasing to menstruate.

bulimia nervosa an illness affecting at least 2 per cent of adolescent women. The woman goes on 'eating binges' at least once a week. Between binges she diets strictly or induces vomiting so that she doesn't put on weight. She might use laxatives to 'clear out the bad food'.

chromosome inherited genetic material that determines the sex of an individual.

colposcopy examination of the vulva using a microscope.

conception this occurs when a man's sperm fertilises a woman's ovum.

contraception the use of hormones, appliances, or 'natural' methods to prevent an unwanted pregnancy and to 'space' the number of children a couple choose to have. Methods include: condom, pill, vaginal diaphragm, IUD, periodic abstinence.

depression a feeling of sadness and that nothing matters any more. The woman doesn't sleep well and might always feel tired.

drug any chemical substance that affects the workings of the body or the mind; some are legal, others are illegal. Drugs include: caffeine, alcohol, tobacco, tranquillisers, cannabis, heroin, cocaine.

dysmenorrhoea crampy pains in the lower part of the abdomen that occur during menstruation.

eating disorder an illness that follows abnormal eating behaviour. The eating disorders are anorexia nervosa, bulimia nervosa, and obesity.

ejaculation the emission of semen from a man's penis.

exercise disorder a condition in which an individual exercises compulsively to the detriment of other aspects of lifestyle.

family planning clinic a clinic, predominantly run by women, where people can obtain contraceptive and other advice in a supportive, friendly environment.

fertilisation occurs when the head of the sperm penetrates the hard shell surrounding the ovum and fuses with the ovum's nucleus.

fetus the unborn baby more than eight weeks after conception.

gender identity the awareness of a person, and the persistence of the awareness, that she is a female (or he is a male).

gender role everything a person does or says to indicate to others (and herself) the degree to which she is a female.

gynaecologist a doctor who specialises in medical problems that relate specifically to women.

heterosexual a person who is sexually and emotionally attracted to members of the opposite sex.

HIV the human immunodeficiency virus that causes AIDS.

homosexual a person who is sexually (and usually emotionally) attracted to a person of her or his own sex. In all other aspects the person is not different from anybody else.

hormones chemical substances made in special body glands, which are secreted into the blood and cause changes in other parts of the body.

incest a sexual assault on a person by a close family member, usually a parent, a brother, an uncle, a grandfather, or a stepfather.

masturbation the self-stimulation of the genitals. In a woman, the stimulation of the clitoral area, usually with her fingers. This produces a warm pleasurable sensation and can lead to orgasm.

menarche the time when the first menstrual period occurs.

menopause the time when the last menstrual period occurs.

menstrual cycle the time from the first day of menstruation till the next menstruation starts.

menstruation the periodic discharge from the uterus of a mixture of blood, tissue fluids, and tiny pieces of the lining of the uterus.

obese a person who is unhealthily overweight (at least a third more than their healthy weight range).

oral sex the activity of a man or woman licking or sucking the genital area of their sexual partner.

orgasm a feeling of intense pleasure that occurs as the climax of sexual intercourse.

ovulation the time during the menstrual cycle when one or other ovary releases an egg.

ovum the egg of the woman, which, when fertilised by a man's sperm, is capable of producing a new individual.

Pap smear a test conducted to find out whether a woman has abnormal cells in her cervix that might lead to cancer.

peer group people of similar age and similar behaviours, habits, or beliefs.

period the most common term for the time when a woman menstruates.

puberty the time when the signs of sexual maturity become visible; for women, the time from the onset of menstruation to full sexual development.

purulent a discharge containing pus.

rape an assault in which a person uses force, or threatens to use force, to have sexual intercourse.

rape crisis centre a place where a rape victim can go to receive medical attention and advice about what to do after the rape.

self-esteem the feeling of being a worthwhile person and having the confidence to deal with life.

semen sperm-rich fluid released by a man's penis at orgasm.

sexual abuse abuse by another person about the victim's sexuality and behaviour. The abuse could be verbal or physical. If it is physical it is sexual assault.

sexual assault physical sexual abuse by another person. Attempted sexual assault includes coercing a person to engage in physical sexual behaviour they do not wish to participate in.

sexual intercourse the sexual activity that involves penetration of a woman's vagina by a man's penis.

sexually transmitted diseases infectious diseases that are always or usually transmitted by close sexual contact. They include: non-gonococcal genital infection, *Chlamydia*, genital herpes, genital warts, gonorrhoea, syphilis, AIDS. The contact can be between the vagina and the penis or the anus and the penis, or might be oral sex.

sperm the male reproductive seed.

standard drink the volume of any alcoholic beverage which contains 10 grams of alcohol.

transsexual a person who feels that their biological sex is wrong, that is, a male who really feels that he should have been a woman, and vice-versa.

ultrasound pictures of the internal organs of the body made by bouncing sound waves off the organs to be examined

vegetarian a person who chooses not to eat meat; strict vegetarians (vegans) do not eat or drink any sort of animal product.

virgin a person who has not participated in sexual intercourse.

Further reading

Abraham, S. & Llewellyn-Jones, D., *Eating Disorders: The Facts*, 5th edn, Oxford University Press, Oxford, 2001.

Bennett, C., *Growing Pains*, Doubleday, Sydney, 1995.? New edition

Guillebaud, J., *The Pill*, 5th edn, Oxford University Press, Oxford, 1997.

Llewellyn-Jones, D., *Everywoman*, 8th edn, Penguin Books, Ringwood (Vic.), 1998.

Llewellyn-Jones, D., *Sexually Transmitted Diseases*, Faber & Faber, London, 1990.

Llewellyn-Jones, D., *Understanding Sexuality*, 3rd edn, Oxford University Press, Melbourne, 1988.

MacKie, R., *Healthy Skin: The Facts*, Oxford University Press, Oxford, 1992.

Index